Tips and Tricks in Fetal Echocardiography

Tips and Tricks in Fetal Echocardiography

Kuldeep Singh MBBS FAUI FICMCH FICMU
Consultant Ultrasonologist
Special Interest in Obstetric Sonology
in Detailed Anomaly Scanning and
Color Doppler for Management and
Gynecological Scanning

Dr Kuldeep's Ultrasound and Color Doppler Clinic
D 80, East of Kailash
New Delhi 110065, India

For Appointments:
Routine call : 09811196613
Level II call : 09811977372
Fetal Echo call : 09911196613

JAYPEE

JAYPEE BROTHERS MEDICAL PUBLISHERS (P) LTD

New Delhi • London • Philadelphia • Panama

Jaypee Brothers Medical Publishers (P) Ltd.

Headquarters

Jaypee Brothers Medical Publishers (P) Ltd.
4838/24, Ansari Road, Daryaganj
New Delhi 110 002, India
Phone: +91-11-43574357
Fax: +91-11-43574314
Email: jaypee@jaypeebrothers.com

Overseas Offices

J.P. Medical Ltd.
83, Victoria Street, London
SW1H 0HW (UK)
Phone: +44-2031708910
Fax: +02-03-0086180
Email: info@jpmedpub.com

Jaypee-Highlights Medical
Publishers Inc.
City of Knowledge, Bld. 237, Clayton
Panama City, Panama
Phone: +507-301-0496
Fax: +507-301-0499
Email: cservice@jphmedical.com

Jaypee Medical Inc.
The Bourse
111, South Independence Mall East
Suite 835, Philadelphia
PA 19106, USA
Phone: + 267-519-9789
Email: joe.rusko@jaypeebrothers.com

Jaypee Brothers Medical
Publishers (P) Ltd.
17/1-B, Babar Road, Block-B
Shaymali, Mohammadpur
Dhaka-1207, Bangladesh
Mobile: +08801912003485
Email: jaypeedhaka@gmail.com

Jaypee Brothers Medical
Publishers (P) Ltd.
Shorakhute
Kathmandu, Nepal
Phone: +00977-9841528578
Email: jaypee.nepal@gmail.com

Website: www.jaypeebrothers.com
Website: www.jaypeedigital.com

Inquiries for bulk sales may be solicited at: jaypee@jaypeebrothers.com

Tips and Tricks in Fetal Echocardiography

First Edition: **2014**

ISBN 978-93-5090-960-7

Printed at: Replika Press Pvt. Ltd.

This book is dedicated
to my parents
Mrs Yoginder Kaur
Mr KJ Singh
who are with God

In Fond
Remembrance of
My Dear Pet Suzi

Preface

With detecting anomalies becoming more challenging and cardiac anomalies on the rise, it becomes essential to know the complete cardiac anatomy evaluation. With a beating heart, it becomes more difficult to evaluate it. For anybody doing ultrasounds, it is the fetal heart which is the most difficult because of change in the fetal position. If a proper methodology is worked on one can confidently say that one is looking at a normal heart though always with a few exceptions of false positive and false negative diagnoses.

With this book providing the basic and simple way of assessing the fetal heart, it should not be difficult in your targetted scan to evaluate the fetal heart.

Kuldeep Singh

Acknowledgments

Thanks to my family Nishu (wife), Jaanvi (daughter) and Jeet (son). My sincere thanks to Shri Jitendar P Vij (Group Chairman) for his confidence, Mr Ankit Vij (Managing Director), Mr Tarun Duneja (Director-Publishing) for his persistence and the team Mr KK Raman (Production Manager), Mr Sunil Kumar Dogra (Production Coordinator), Ms Samina Khan (PA to Director-Publishing), Mrs Yashu Kapoor (Typesetter), Mr Manoj Pahuja (Graphic Designer) and Mr Ashwani Kumar (Proofreader) of M/s Jaypee Brothers Medical Publishers (P) Ltd, New Delhi, India.

Thanks to my seniors, well-wishers and colleagues.

Contents

1

Introduction

1. Congenital heart defects are one of the common and often lethal congenital anomalies, having an estimated incidence of approximately 1% of all live births.
2. A screening four-chamber view of the heart could detect only 50 to 60% of cardiac malformations. Visualization of the right and the left ventricular outflow tracts, performed properly increases the sensitivity of detecting defects in the range of approximately 75%.
3. Other real-time views (short axis, oblique views, sagittal views) when combined with color-flow mapping, pulsed Doppler, M-mode echocardiography with 3D/4D (STIC) are needed to obtain a complete study for understanding more complex cardiac malformations.

2

Prerequisites

1. Variable frequency high-resolution real-time equipment using linear, curved, or sector transducers can be used for fetal echocardiography. It is important to use transducer frequencies as high as possible, in the range of 5 to 8 MHz. Image magnification and cine loops for instantaneous playback of information are recommended. Digital storage of information in real time, either with software available within the ultrasound equipment or a separate attached video recorder, is helpful for review of the study and to further analyze data frame by frame to elucidate some of the more subtle findings.
2. Although useful, there may be limitations, especially during the second trimester, when gray-scale imaging can be limited by fetal position, maternal adipose tissue, or abdominal wall scar from previous abdominal or pelvic surgery.

3

Salient Features

A normal fetal heart should:

- Be in the fetal thorax
- Be and point to the left side
- Be of normal size
- Have four chambers, two atria and two ventricles
- Have six veins, two caval and four pulmonary veins
- Have two arteries, aorta and pulmonary artery
- Have two atrioventricular valves
- Have an atrial septum with a gap in the foramen ovale
- Have an interventricular septum with no gap.

4

Fetal Visceral Situs

1. There are three types of visceral situs—situs solitus, situs inversus, and situs ambiguous. Situs solitus is the normal arrangement of vessels and organs within the body. Situs inversus denotes a mirror-image arrangement of organs and vessels to situs solitus and is associated with a slight increase in the incidence of complex congenital heart disease.
2. The most common method for the determining fetal situs is the position of the stomach and heart in the abdomen and chest, respectively.
3. Attention should also be paid to the position of the aorta and inferior vena cava below the diaphragm and the presence of a gallbladder.

1. There are three types of visceral situs—situs solitus, situs inversus, and situs ambiguous. Situs solitus is the normal arrangement of vessels and organs within the body (Fig. 1). Situs inversus denotes a mirror-image arrangement of organs and vessels to situs solitus and is associated with a slight increase in the incidence of complex congenital heart disease.

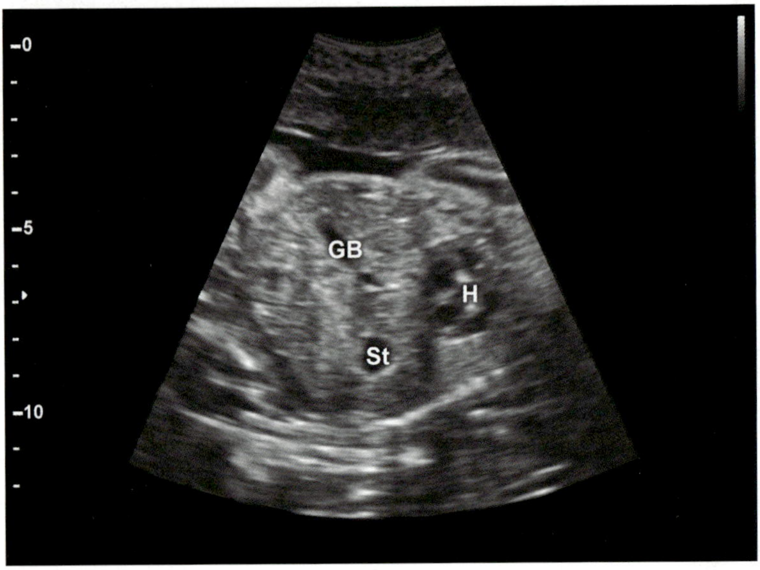

Fig. 1

2. The most common method for the determining fetal situs is the position of the stomach and heart in the abdomen and chest, respectively (Fig. 2).

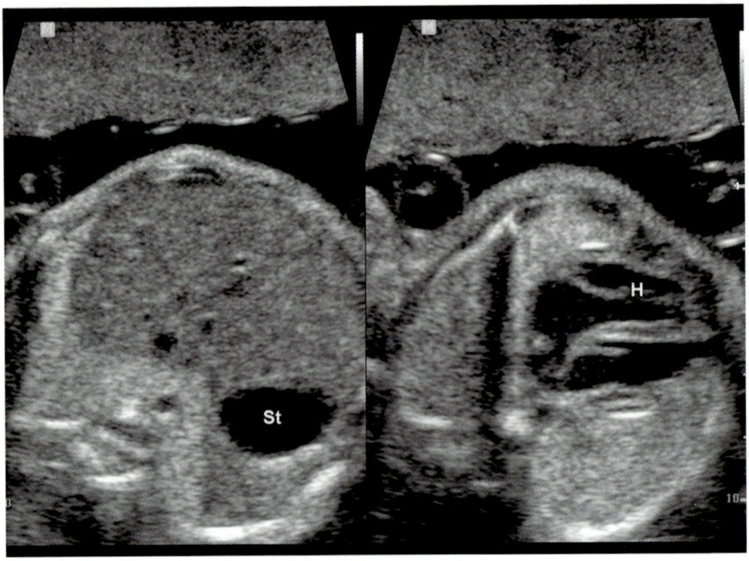

Fig. 2

3. Attention should also be paid to the position of the aorta and inferior vena cava below the diaphragm (Fig. 3A) and the presence of a gallbladder (Fig. 3B).

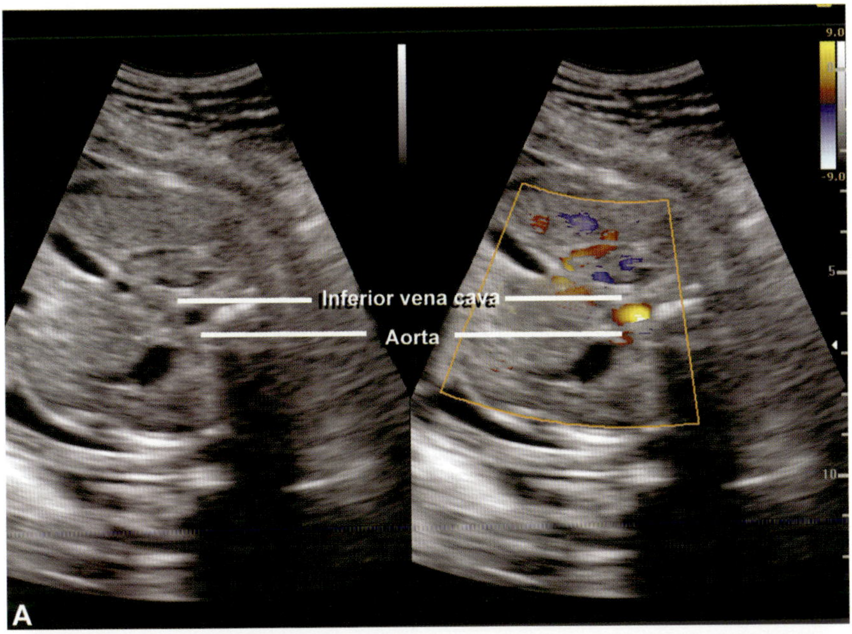

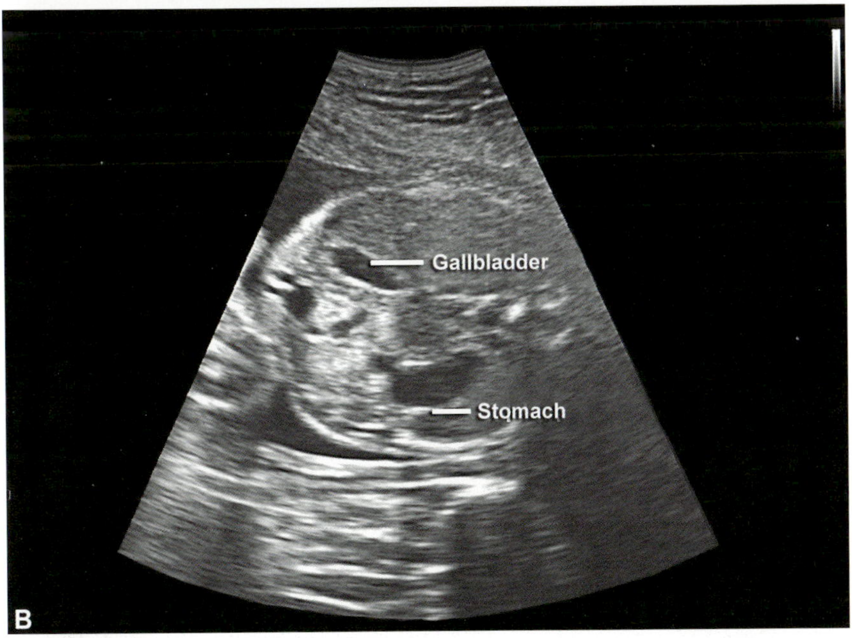

Figs 3A and B

5

Size

1. The fetal heart occupies approximately one-third of the thoracic cavity in the center (Fig. 1).
2. Fetal cardiac dimensions can be assessed by measuring the linear cardiac size/diameter in the four-chamber view (Fig. 2A) in respect to the thoracic size/diameter from the spine to the anterior thoracic wall (Fig. 2B) (cardio-thoracic ratio).
3. Fetal cardiac dimensions can also be assessed by measuring the ratio of cardiac circumference or area (Fig. 3A) to the chest circumference or area obtained at the level of the four-chamber view (Fig. 3B).

1. The fetal heart occupies approximately one-third of the thoracic cavity in the center (Fig. 1).

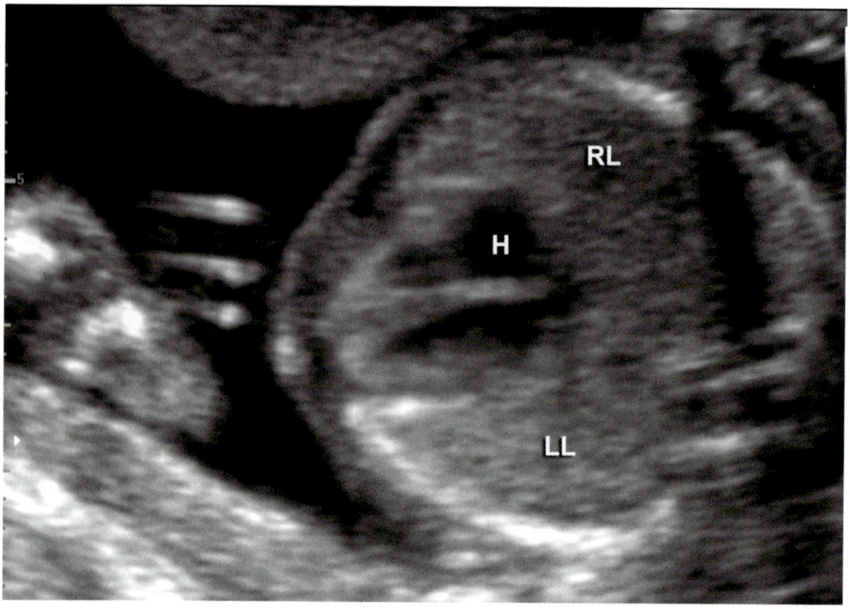

Fig. 1

2. Fetal cardiac dimensions can be assessed by measuring the linear cardiac size/diameter in the four-chamber view (Fig. 2A) in respect to the thoracic size/diameter from the spine to the anterior thoracic wall (Fig. 2B) (cardio-thoracic ratio).

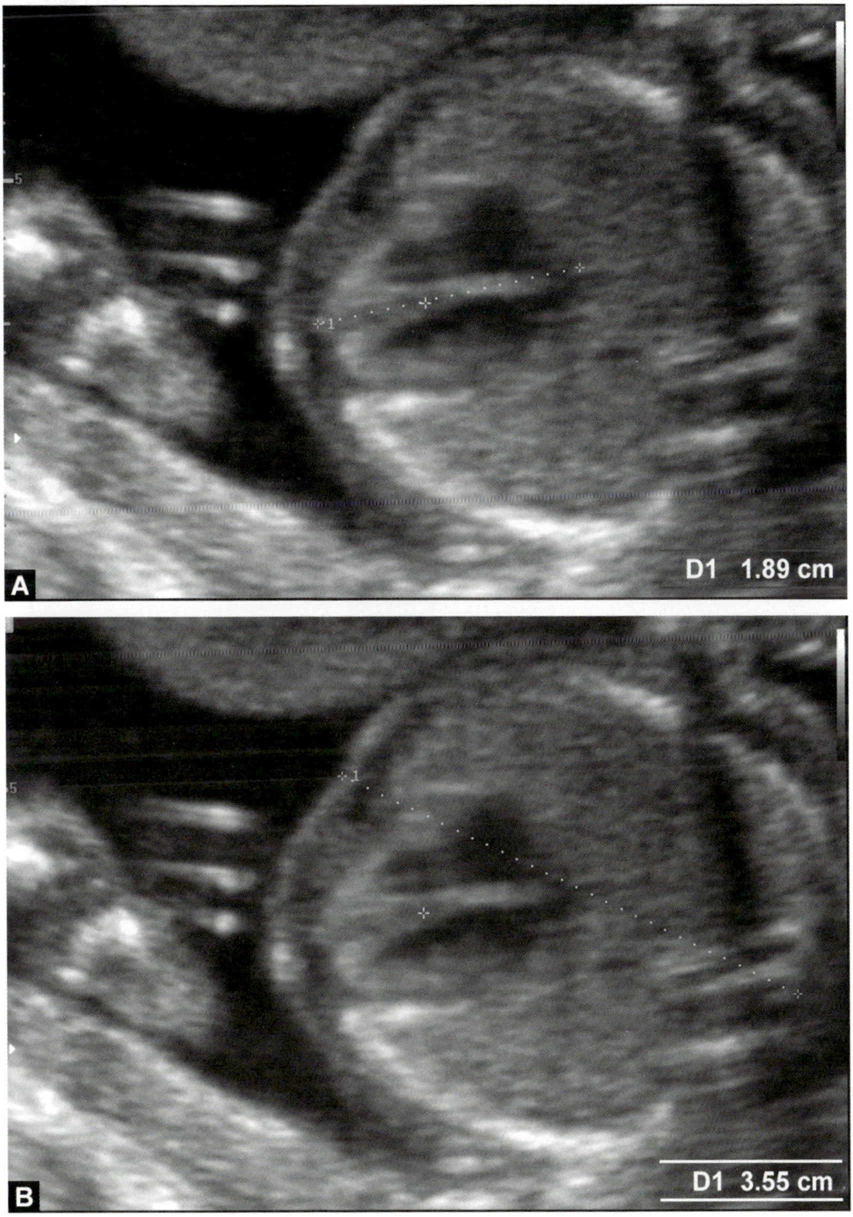

Figs 2A and B

3. Fetal cardiac dimensions can also be assessed by measuring the ratio of cardiac circumference or area (Fig. 3A) to the chest circumference or area obtained at the level of the four-chamber view (Fig. 3B).

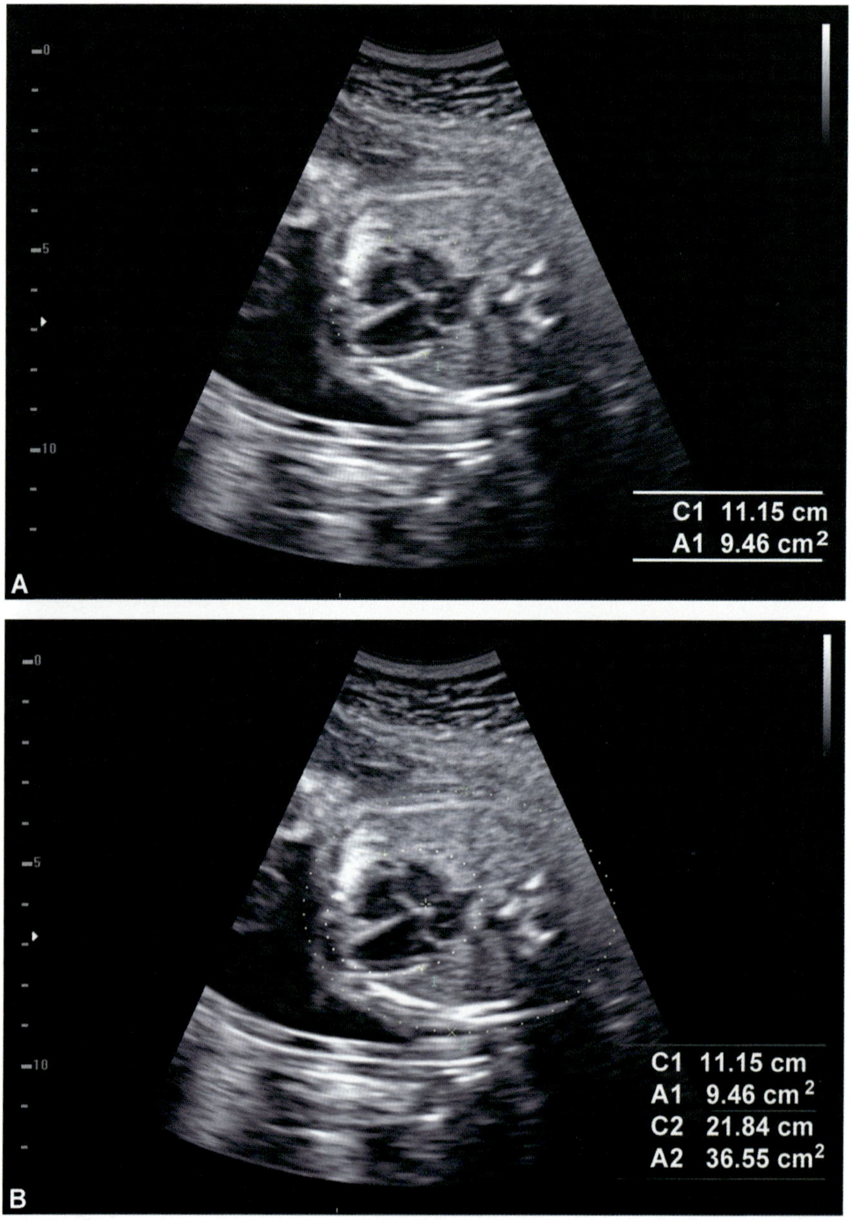

Figs 3A and B

6

Axis

1. The fetal cardiac axis is measured by obtaining a transverse view of the chest at the level of the four-chamber view plane of the heart (Fig. 1).
2. A line is traced from the spine to the anterior chest wall (Fig. 2).
3. The cardiac axis is measured by the angle that the interventricular septum makes with the line from spine to anterior chest wall (Fig. 3).
4. Normal cardiac axis lies at a 45-degree angle to the left of the midline (Fig. 4).

1. The fetal cardiac axis is measured by obtaining a transverse view of the chest at the level of the four-chamber view plane of the heart (Fig. 1).

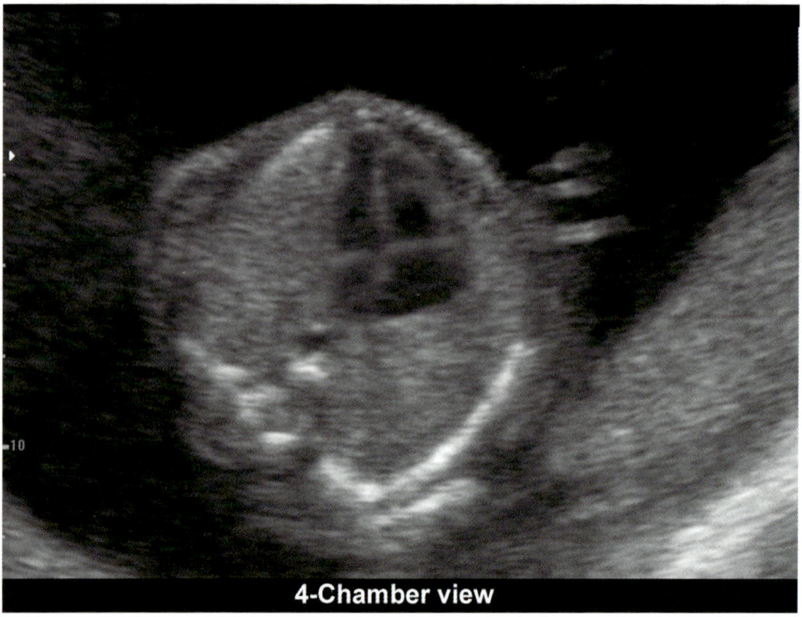

Fig. 1

2. A line is traced from the spine to the anterior chest wall (Fig. 2).

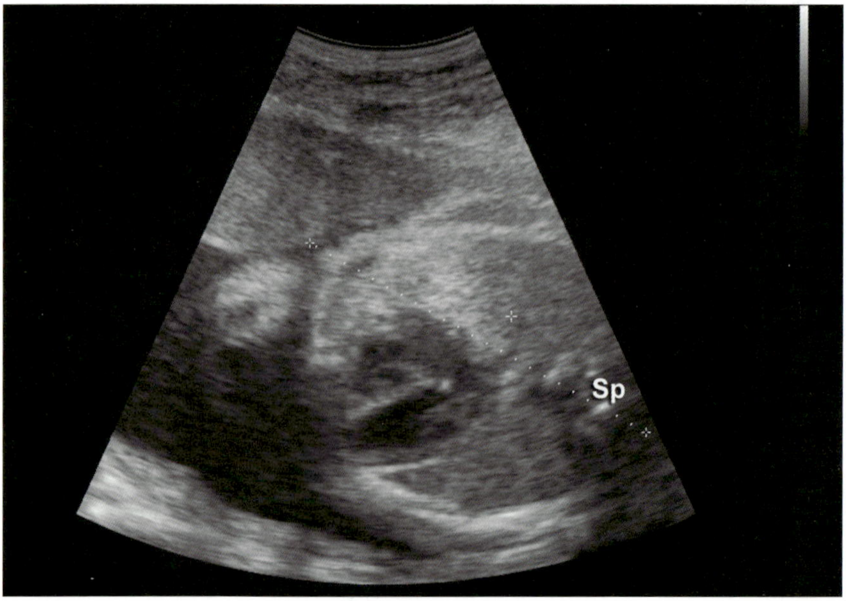

Fig. 2

3. The cardiac axis is measured by the angle that the interventricular septum makes with the line from spine to anterior chest wall (Fig. 3).

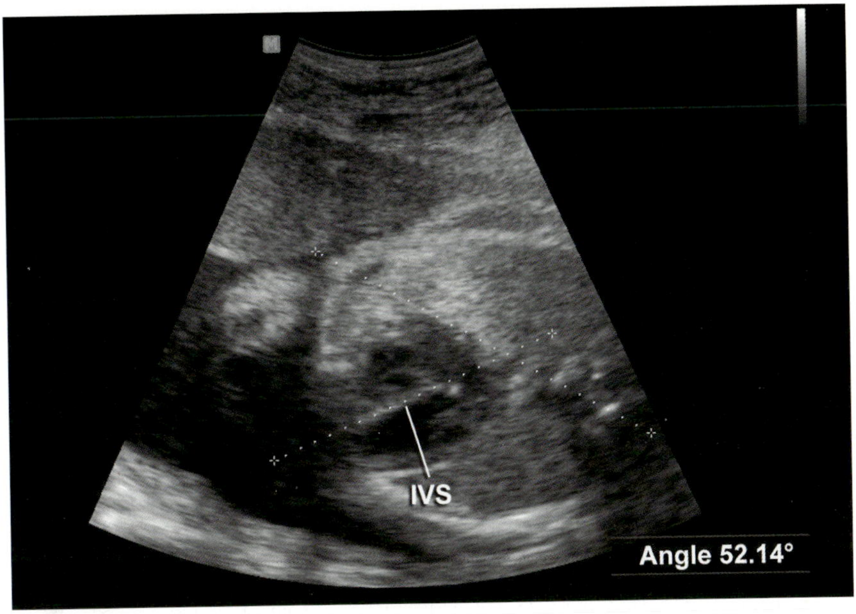

Fig. 3

4. Normal cardiac axis lies at a 45-degree angle to the left of the midline (Fig. 4).

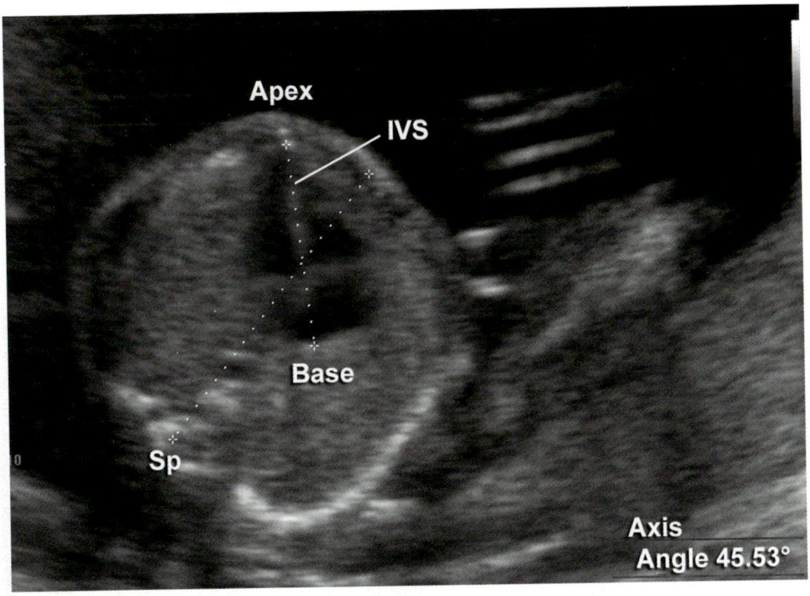

Fig. 4

7

Cardiac Anatomy

A. Caval Veins
   i. Superior Vena Cava
   ii. Inferior Vena Cava
B. Right Atrium
C. Tricuspid Valve
D. Right Ventricle
E. Pulmonary Artery
F. Pulmonary Veins
G. Left Atrium
H. Mitral/Bicuspid Valve
I. Left Ventricle
J. Aorta
K. Foramen Ovale
L. Interventricular Septum

CAVAL VEINS

Superior Vena Cava

1. The superior vena cava (SVC) enters the right atrium anteriorly.
2. The superior vena cava (SVC) is also seen as the lateral most vessel in the 3 vessel view.

Inferior Vena Cava

1. The inferior vena cava (IVC) enters into the right atrium from the inferior aspect at its lowest part, near the interatrial septum.
2. The Eustachian valve, which is a flap, is located at the opening of the inferior vena cava.
3. The inferior vena cava in its longitudinal section is seen on the right side of the fetal aorta.

Superior Vena Cava

1. The superior vena cava (SVC) enters the right atrium anteriorly (Fig. 1).

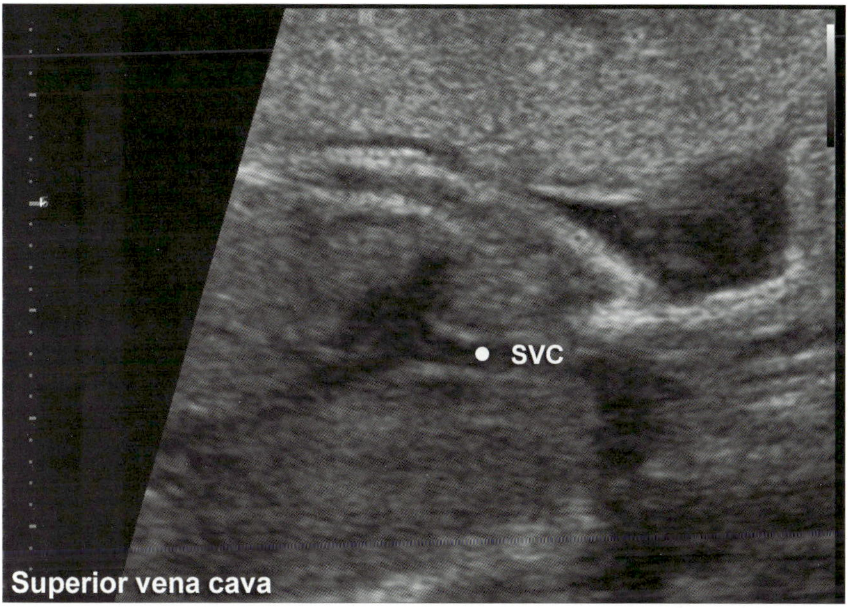

Fig. 1

2. The superior vena cava (SVC) is also seen as the lateral most vessel in the 3 vessel view (Fig. 2).

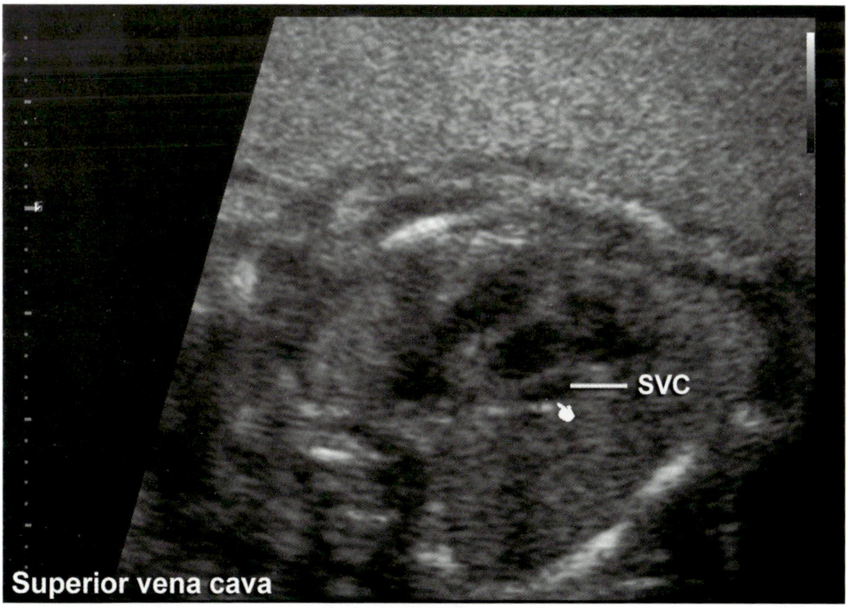

Fig. 2

Inferior Vena Cava

1. The inferior vena cava (IVC) enters into the right atrium from the inferior aspect at its lowest part, near the interatrial septum (Figs 3A to C).

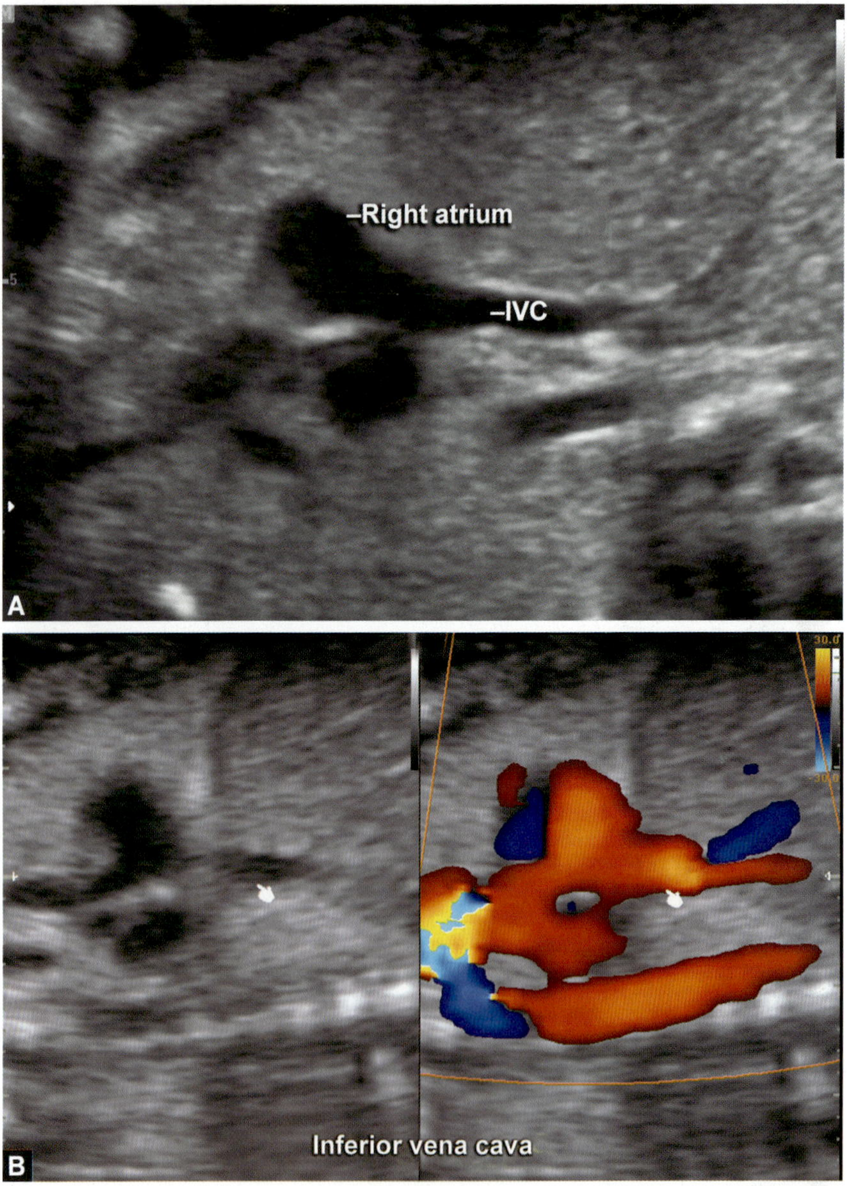

Figs 3A and B

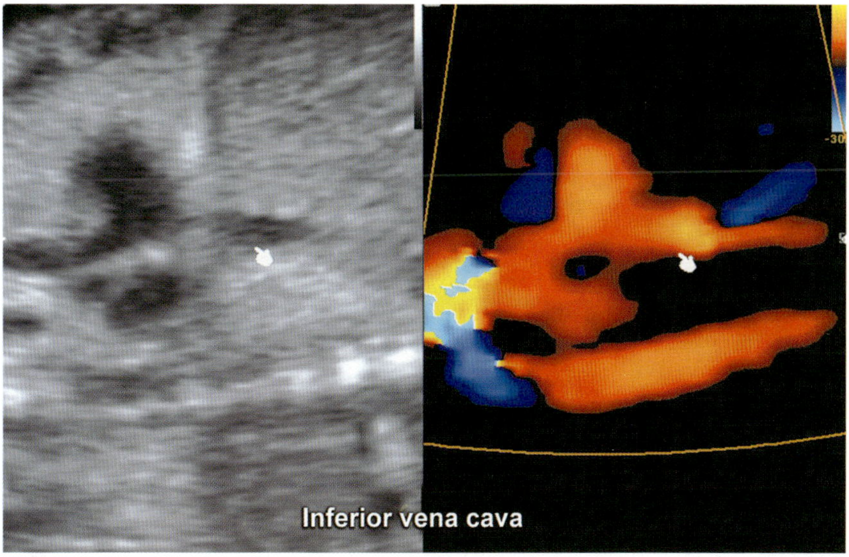

Fig. 3C

2. The Eustachian valve, which is a flap, is located at the opening of the inferior vena cava (Figs 4A to C).

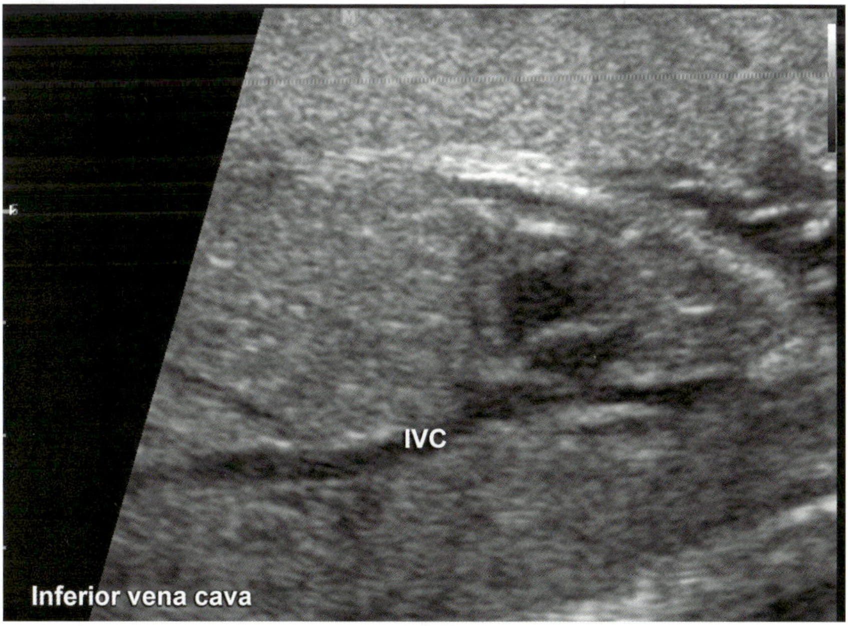

Fig. 4A

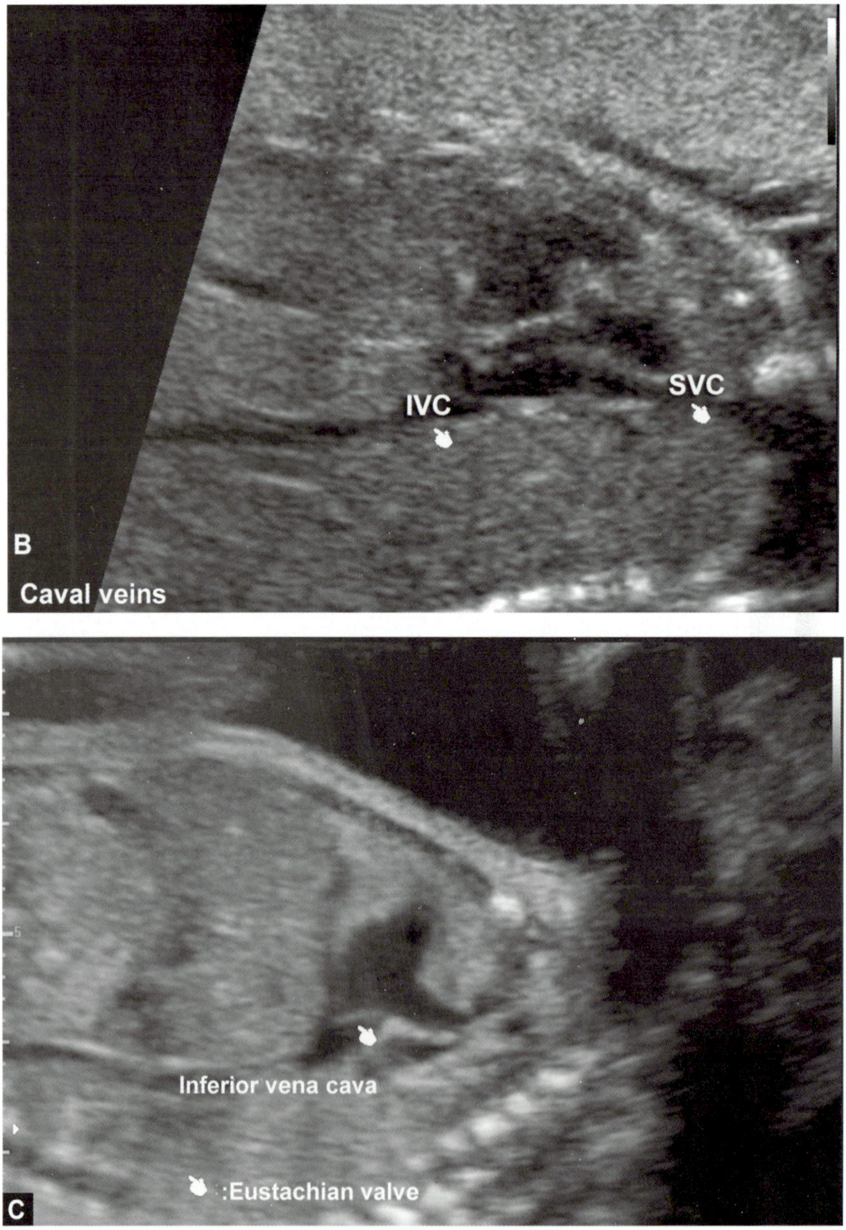

Figs 4B and C

3. The inferior vena cava (IVC) in its longitudinal section is seen on the right side of the fetal aorta (Fig. 5).

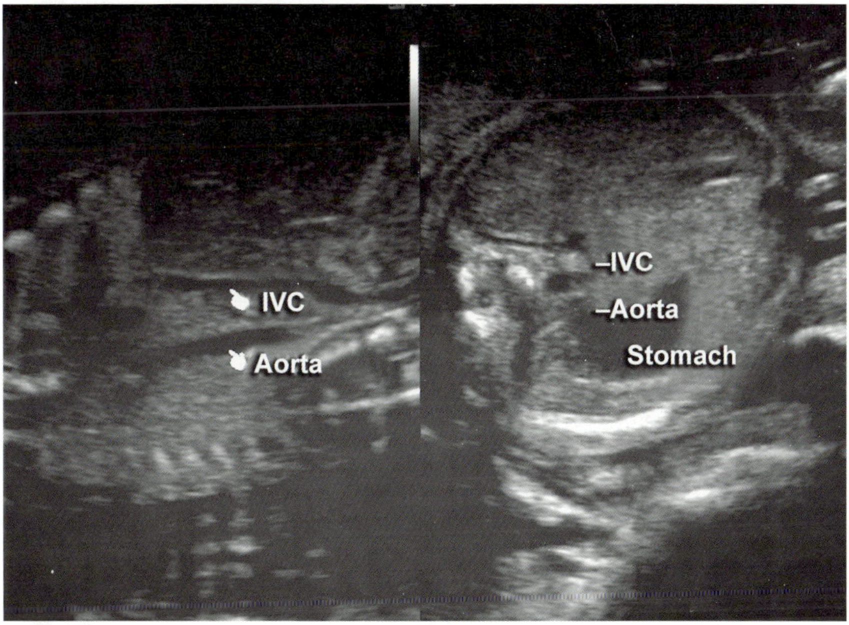

Fig. 5

RIGHT ATRIUM

1. The right atrium is located anteriorly and to the right of the left atrium.
2. The inferior vena cava (IVC) enters into the right atrium from the inferior aspect at its lowest part, near the interatrial septum.
3. The superior vena cava (SVC) enters the right atrium anteriorly.
4. The right atrial appendage is seen as the reverse hammock sign formed by the caval veins and the right atrium. This is pyramidal in shape with a broad base.
5. The atrial septum separates the two atria. The septum primum and secundum form the atrial septum.
6. Blood flows from the right atrium to the left atrium via the foramen ovale.
7. Blood also flows from the right atrium to the right ventricle via the tricuspid valve.

1. The right atrium is located anteriorly and to the right of the left atrium (Fig. 6).

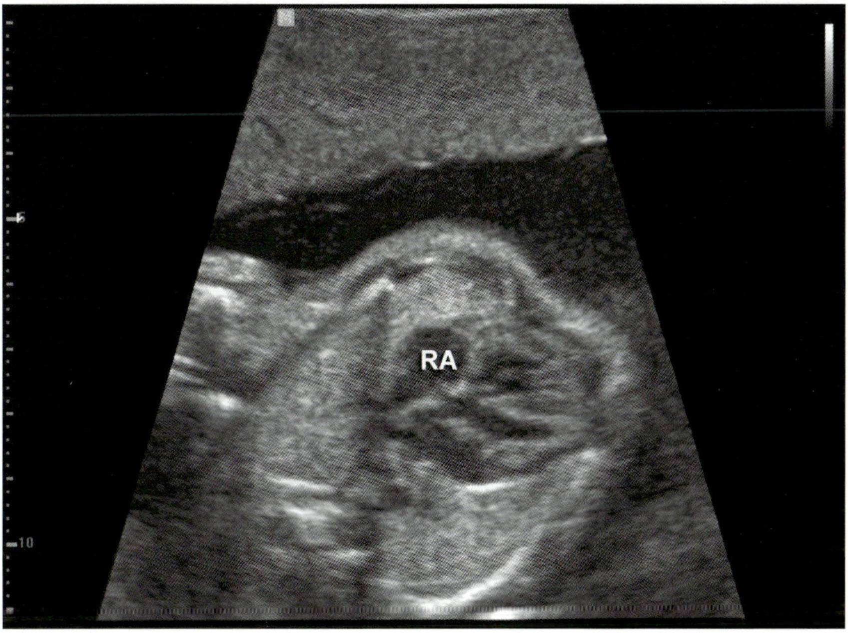

Fig. 6

2. The inferior vena cava (IVC) enters into the right atrium (RA) from the inferior aspect at its lowest part, near the interatrial septum (Fig. 7).

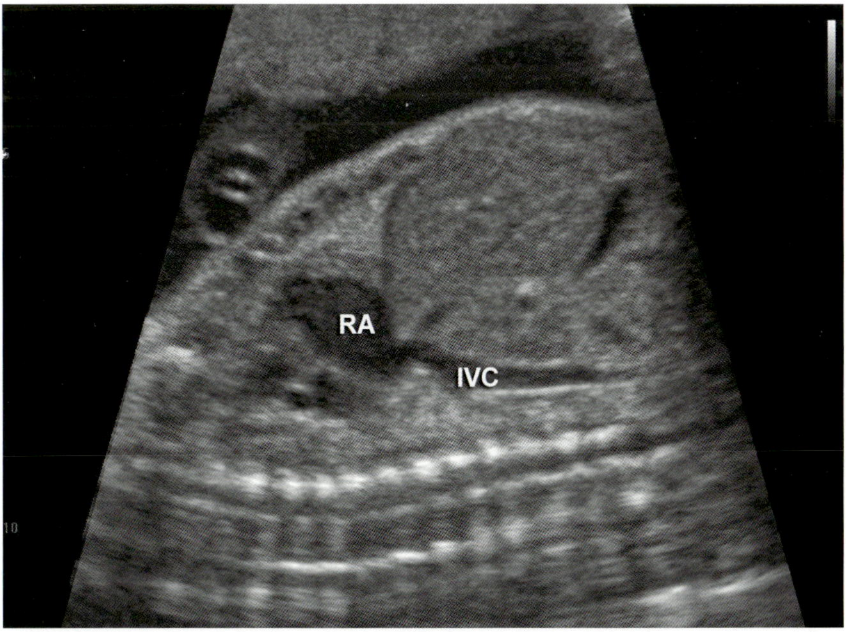

Fig. 7

3. The superior vena cava (SVC) enters the right atrium (RA) anteriorly (Fig. 8).

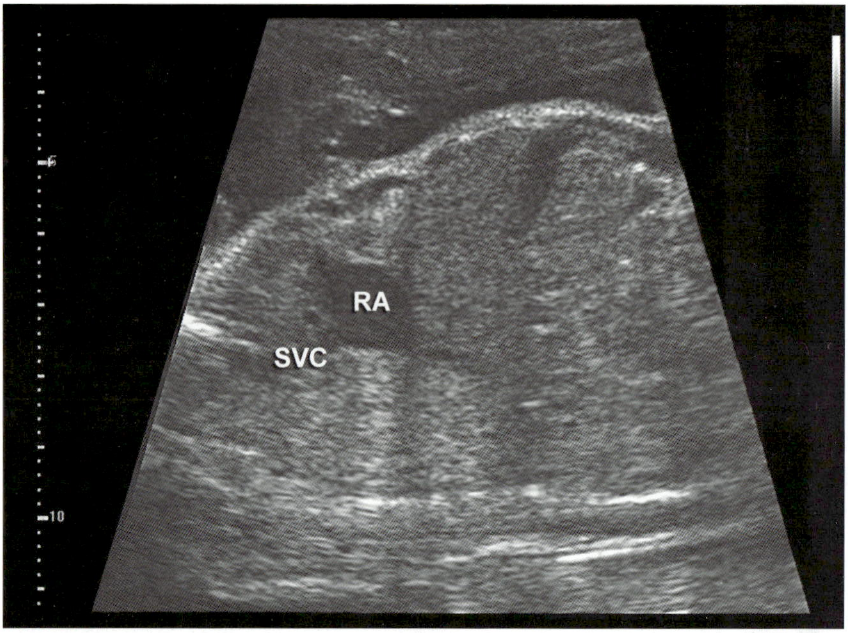

Fig. 8

4. The right atrial appendage is seen as the reverse hammock sign formed by the caval veins and the right atrium. This is pyramidal in shape with a broad base (Fig. 9).

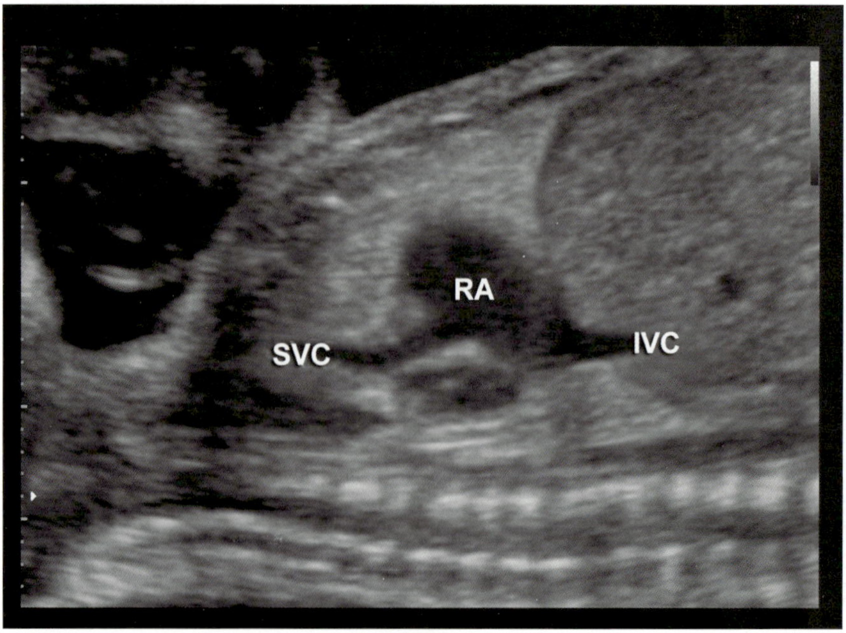

Fig. 9

5. The atrial septum separates the two atria. The septum primum and secundum form the atrial septum (Fig. 10).

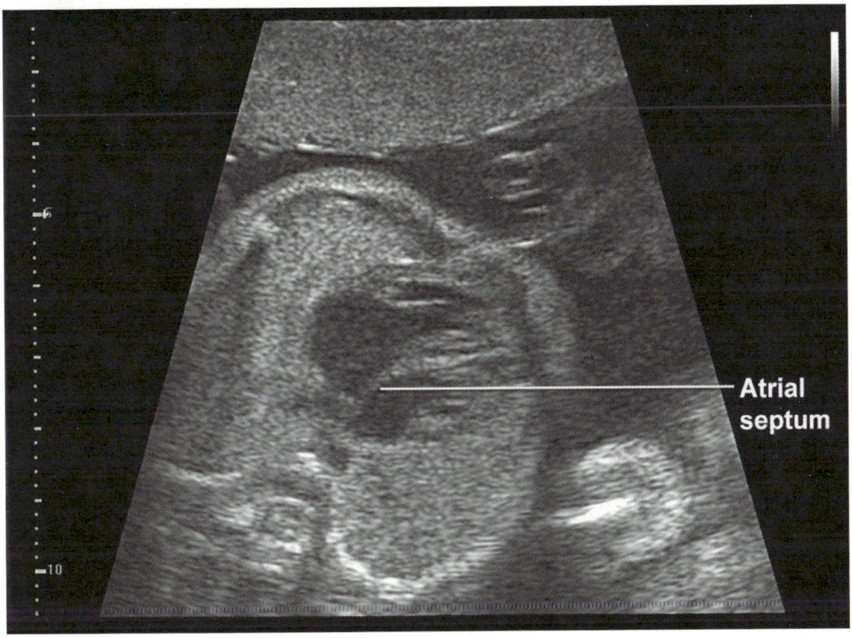

Fig. 10

6. Blood flows from the right atrium to the left atrium via the foramen ovale (Fig. 11).

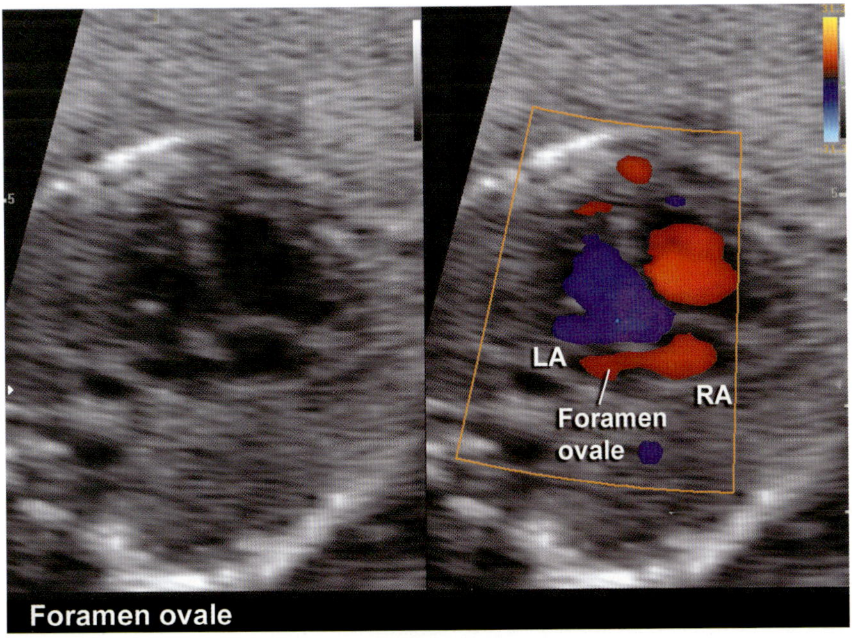

Fig. 11

7. Blood also flows from the right atrium to the right ventricle via the tricuspid valve (Fig. 12).

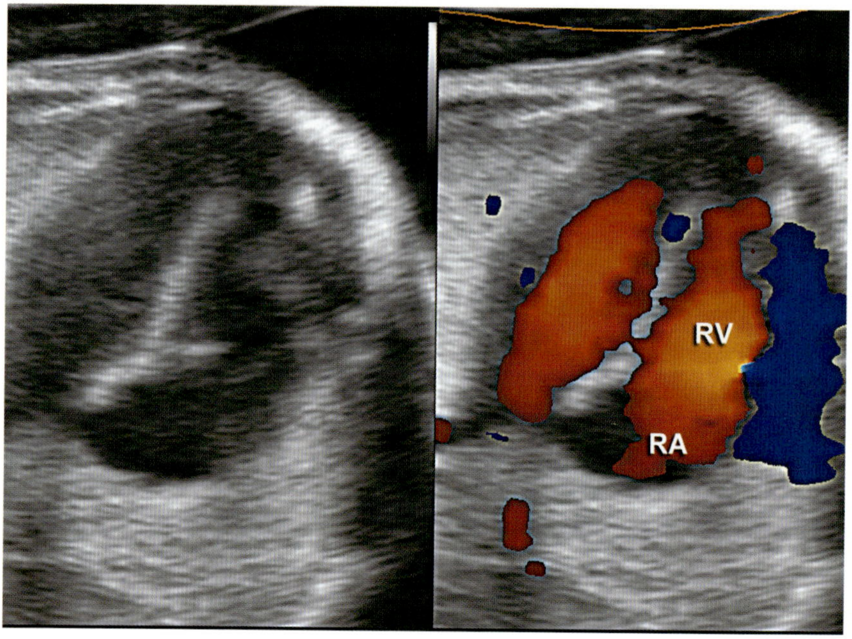

Fig. 12

TRICUSPID

1. The tricuspid or the right atrioventricular valve is located between the right atrium and right ventricle.
2. The tricuspid valve inserts more apically (near to cardiac apex) than the mitral valve on the interventricular septum. This anatomic finding helps in determining ventricular situs and in recognizing atrioventricular canal abnormalities.
3. The tricuspid valve does not allow the blood from flowing back into the right atrium from the right ventricle during ventricular systole.

1. The tricuspid or the right atrioventricular valve is located between the right atrium and right ventricle (Figs 13A and B).

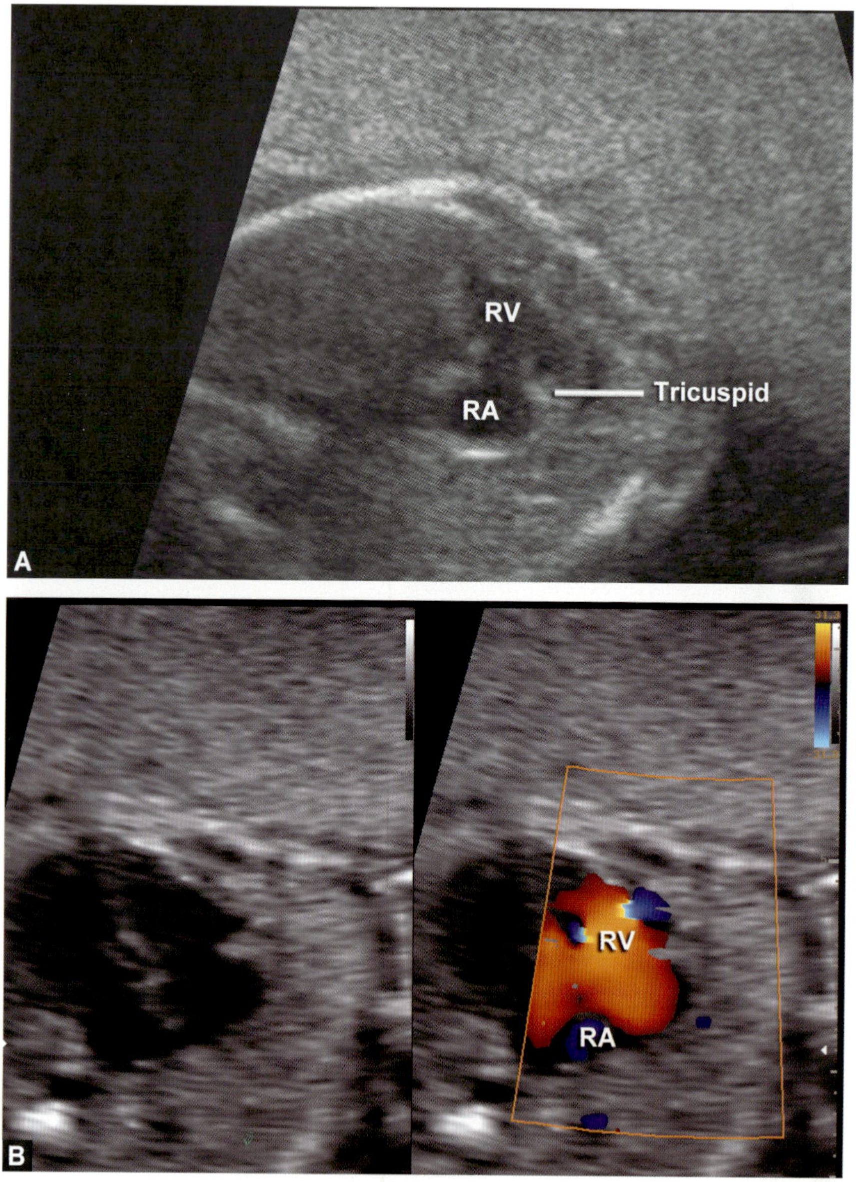

Figs 13A and B

2. The tricuspid valve inserts more apically (near to cardiac apex) than the mitral valve on the interventricular septum. This anatomic finding helps in determining ventricular situs and in recognizing atrioventricular canal abnormalities (Fig. 14).

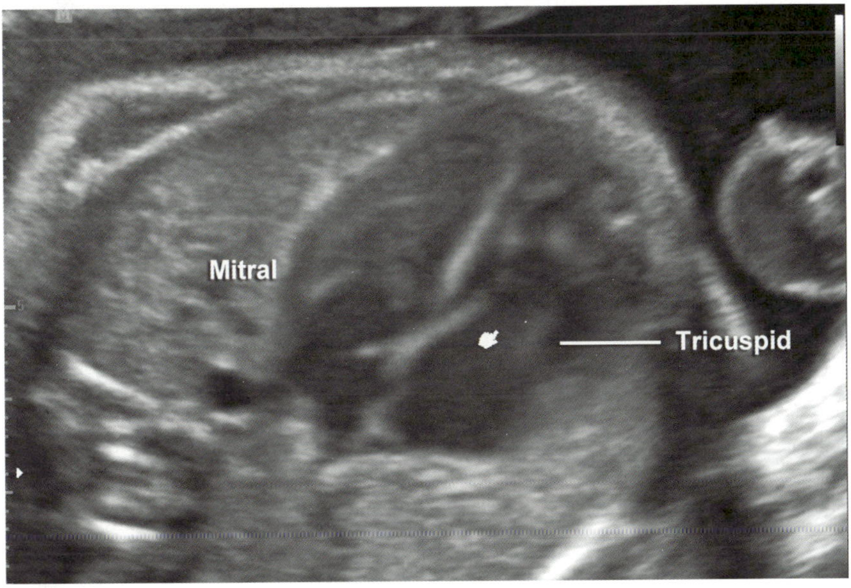

Fig. 14

3. The tricuspid valve does not allow the blood from flowing back into the right atrium from the right ventricle during ventricular systole (Fig. 15).

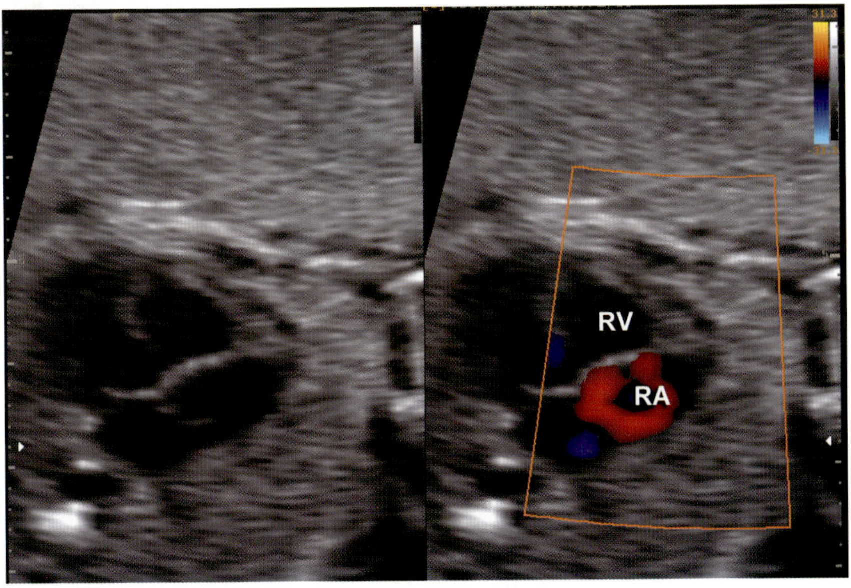

Fig. 15

RIGHT VENTRICLE

1. The right ventricle (RV) is the anterior most cardiac chamber, anatomically located behind the sternum.
2. At the apex of the right ventricle is the moderator band which is a coarse trabeculation occupying the apical portion.
3. The right ventricle receives blood from the right atrium via the tricuspid valve.
4. Blood flows out from the right ventricle through the pulmonary artery (PA).

1. The right ventricle (RV) is the anterior most cardiac chamber, anatomically located behind the sternum (Fig. 16).

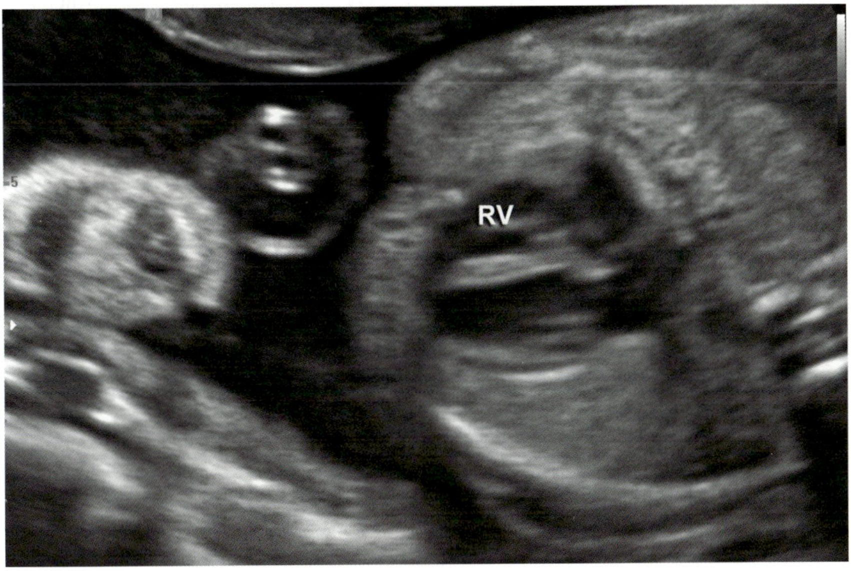

Fig. 16

2. At the apex of the right ventricle is the moderator band which is a coarse trabeculation occupying the apical portion (Fig. 17).

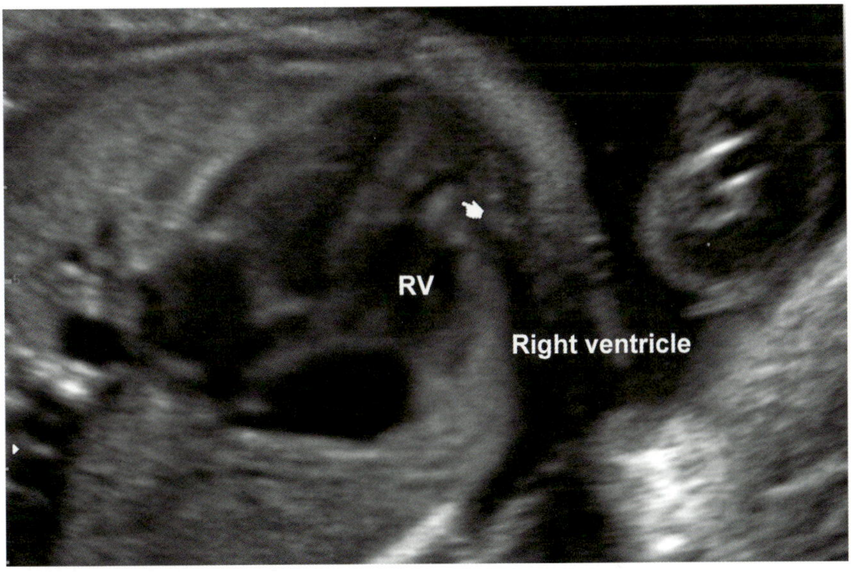

Fig. 17

3. The right ventricle receives blood from the right atrium via the tricuspid valve (Fig. 18).

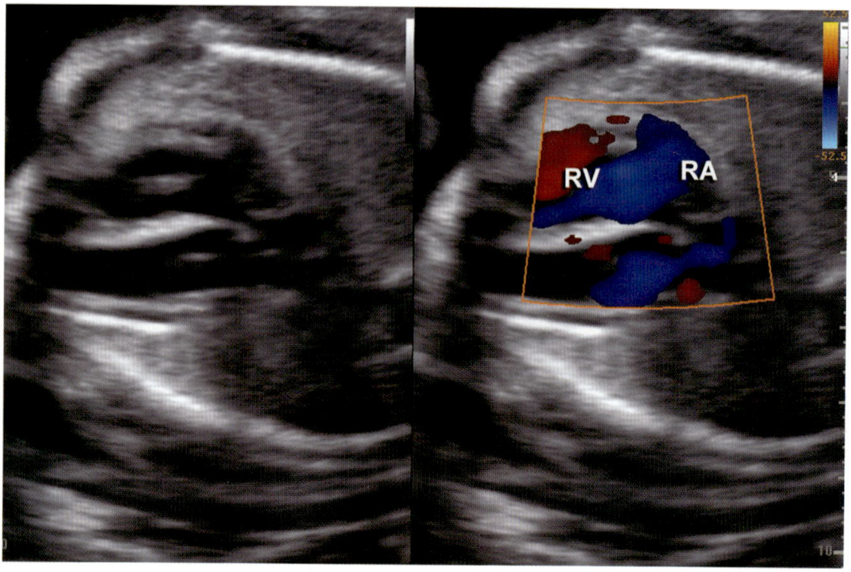

Fig. 18

4. Blood flows out from the right ventricle through the pulmonary artery (Figs 19A and B).

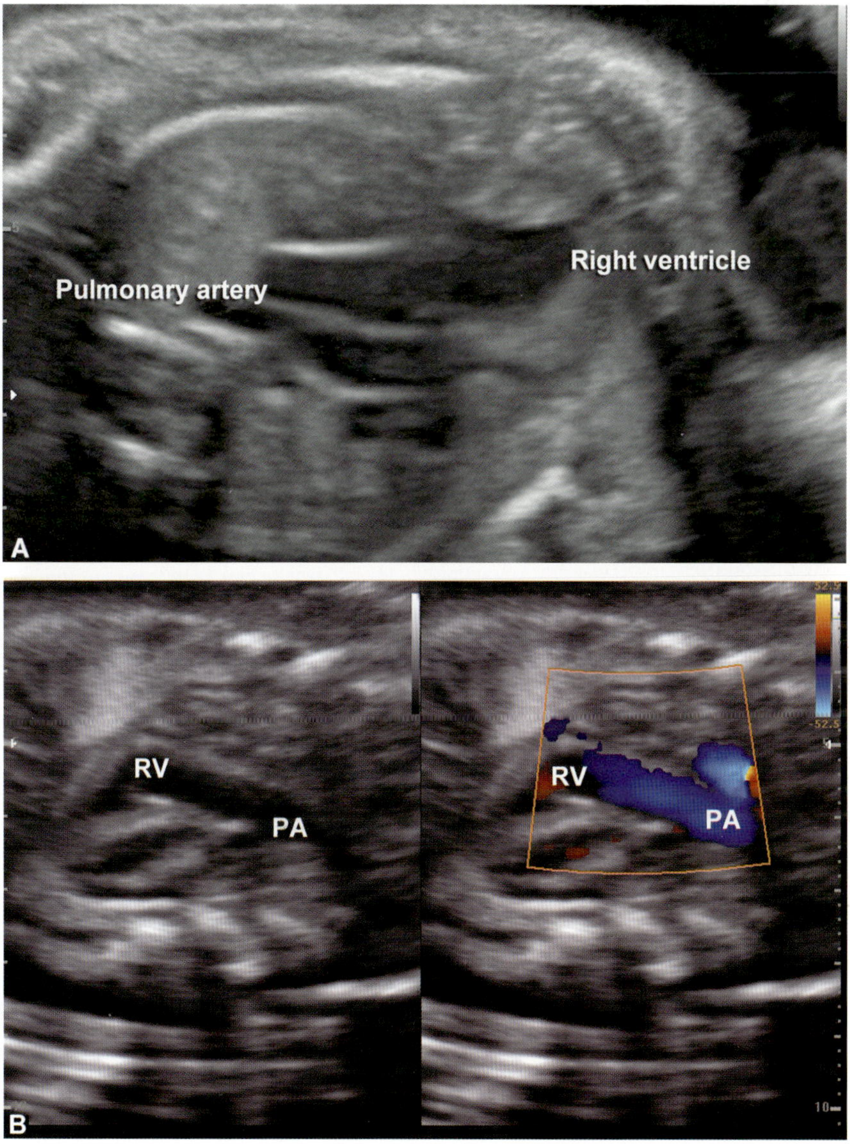

Figs 19A and B

PULMONARY ARTERY

1. The pulmonary artery arises from the right ventricle (RV) in the anterior aspect of the heart.
2. It crosses over the aorta and then points toward the fetal left shoulder after emerging from the right ventricle.
3. The pulmonary artery divides into the right and left pulmonary arteries and the ductus arteriosus.
4. The ductus arteriosus connects with the descending aorta.
5. The pulmonary artery dividing into the right and left pulmonary arteries is an important anatomic landmark that differentiates it from the ascending aorta.
6. The right pulmonary artery originates at a right angle from the pulmonary artery and crosses under the aortic arch, superior to the roof of the left atrium and behind the superior vena cava.
7. During right ventricular diastole, blood is prevented from flowing back into the ventricle by the pulmonary semilunar valve.

1. The pulmonary artery arises from the right ventricle (RV) in the anterior aspect of the heart (Fig. 20).

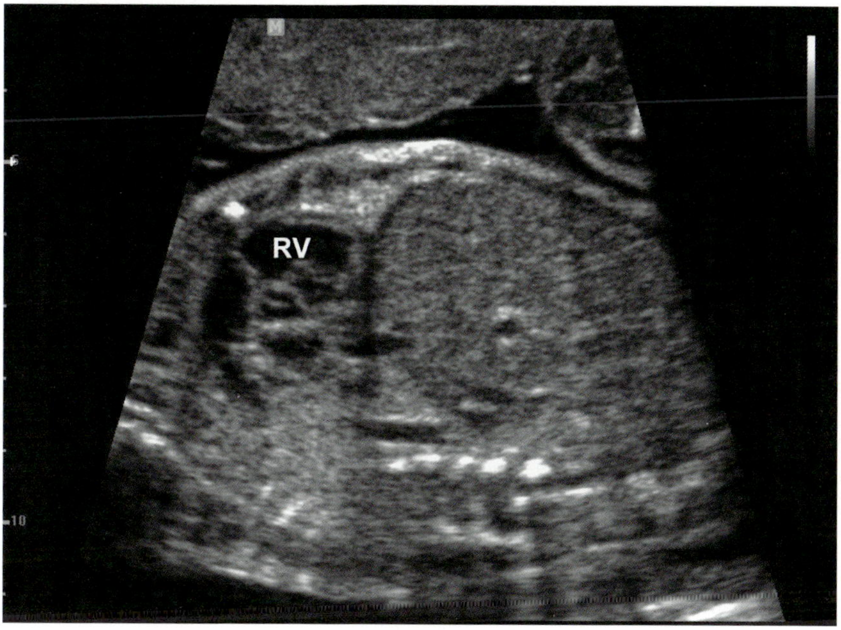

Fig. 20

2. It crosses over the aorta and then points toward the fetal left shoulder after emerging from the right ventricle (Fig. 21).

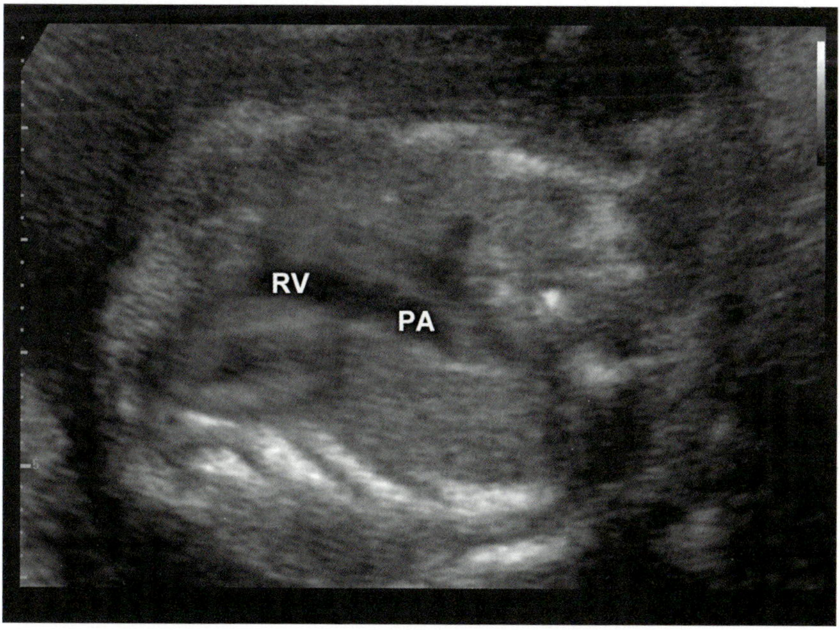

Fig. 21

3. The pulmonary artery divides into the right and left pulmonary arteries and the ductus arteriosus (DA) (Fig. 22).

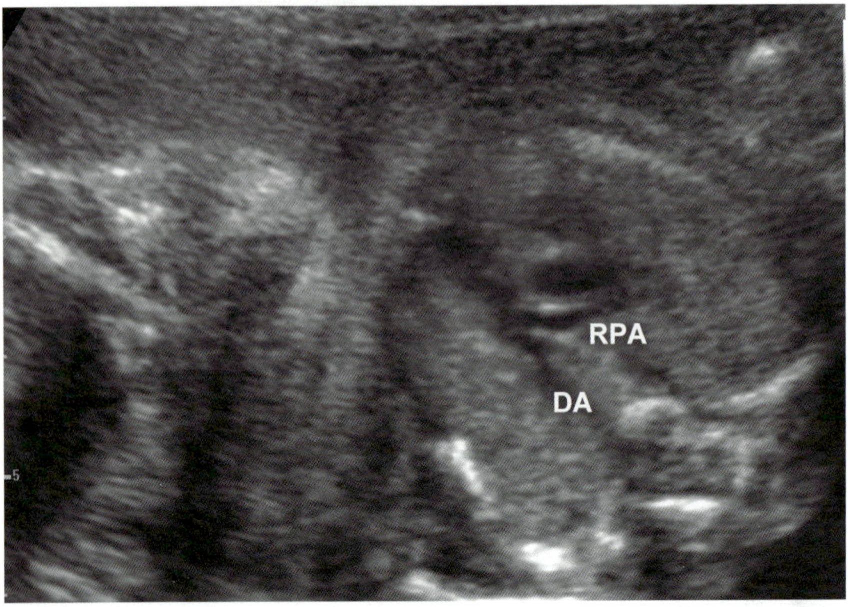

Fig. 22

4. The ductus arteriosus connects with the descending aorta (DAo) (Fig. 23).

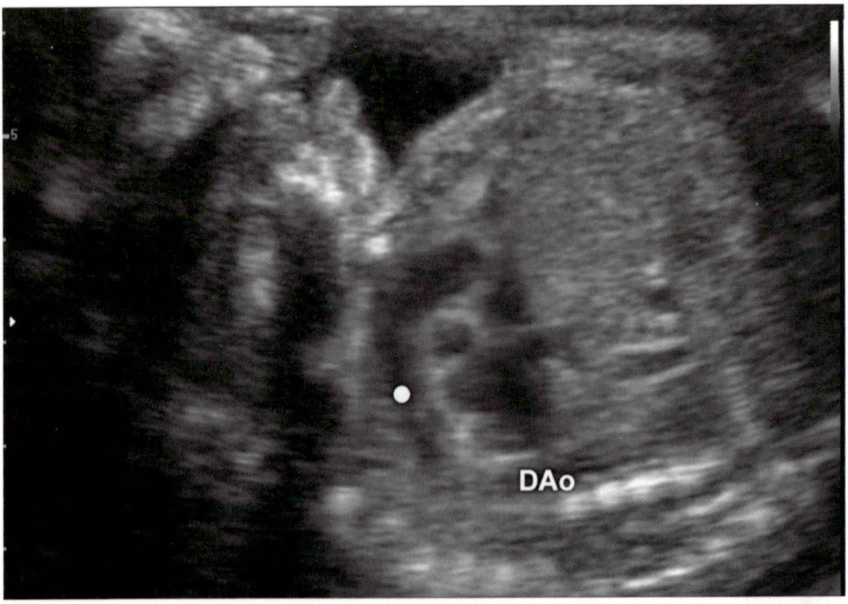

Fig. 23

5. The pulmonary artery dividing into the right and left pulmonary arteries is an important anatomic landmark that differentiates it from the ascending aorta (Fig. 24).

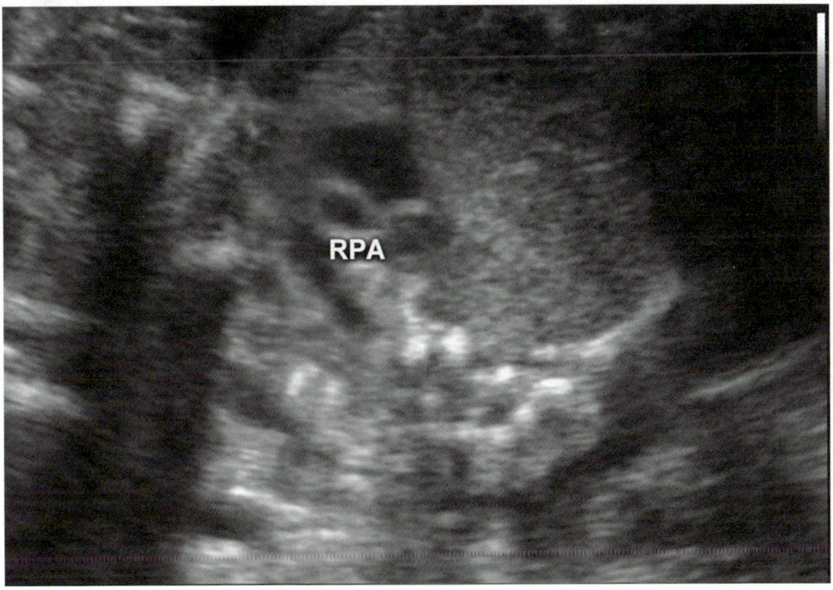

Fig. 24

6. The right pulmonary artery (RPA) originates at a right angle from the pulmonary artery and crosses under the aortic arch, superior to the roof of the left atrium and behind the superior vena cava (Fig. 25).

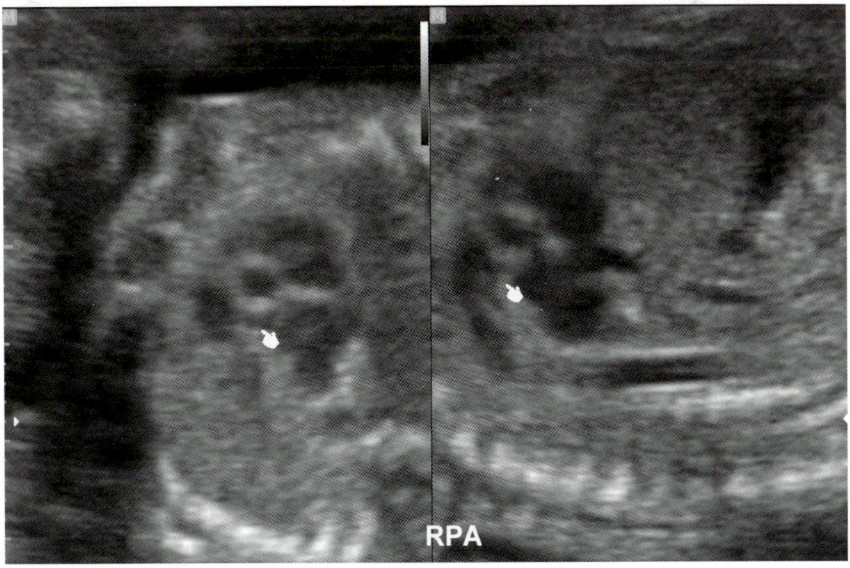

Fig. 25

7. During right ventricular (RV) diastole, blood is prevented from flowing back into the ventricle by the pulmonary semilunar valve (Fig. 26).

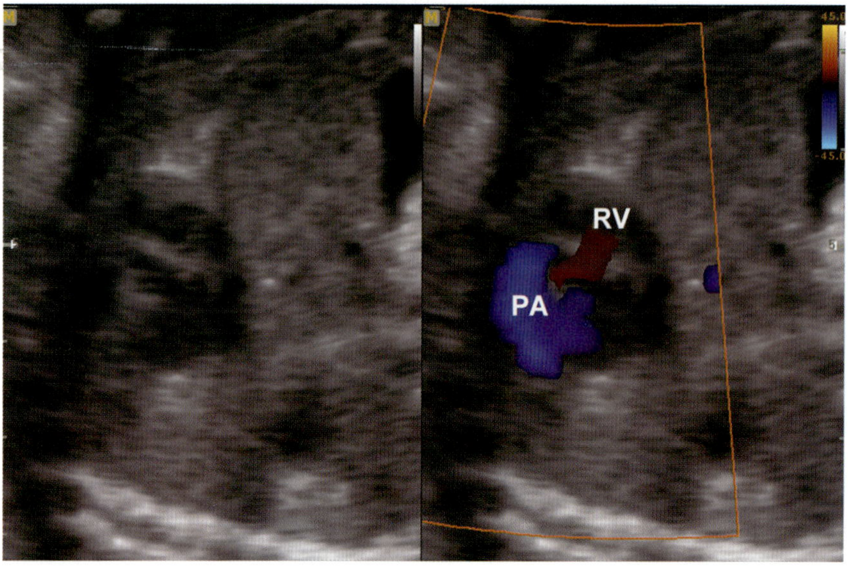

Fig. 26

PULMONARY VEINS

1. The left atrium receives the right and left pulmonary veins.
2. A total of four pulmonary veins, a superior and an inferior pair enter the left atrium on its upper posterolateral surface. At the level of the four-chamber view, only two of the four pulmonary veins are seen as linear openings in the posterior wall of the left atrium.

1. The left atrium (LA) receives the right and left pulmonary veins (Figs 27A and B).

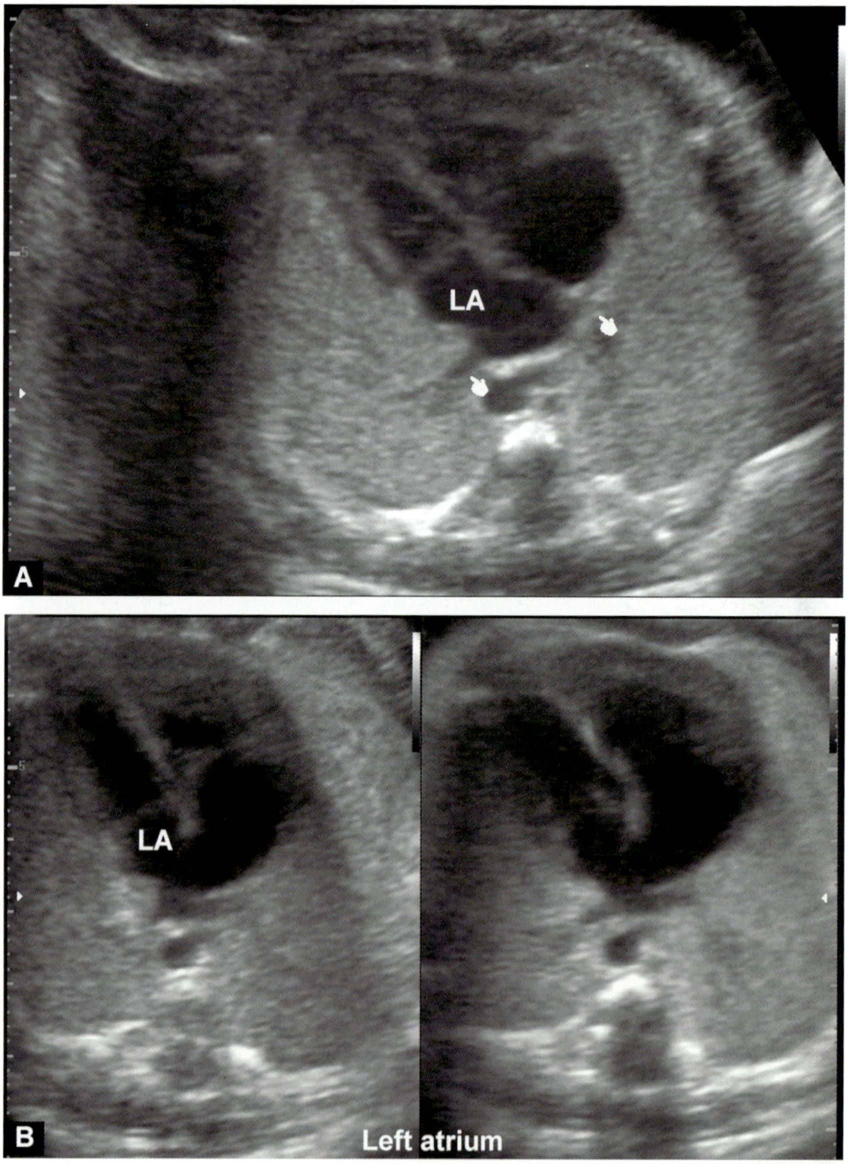

Figs 27A and B

2. A total of four pulmonary veins, a superior and an inferior pair enter the left atrium (LA) on its upper posterolateral surface. At the level of the four-chamber view, only two of the four pulmonary veins are seen as linear openings in the posterior wall of the left atrium (Figs 28A and B).

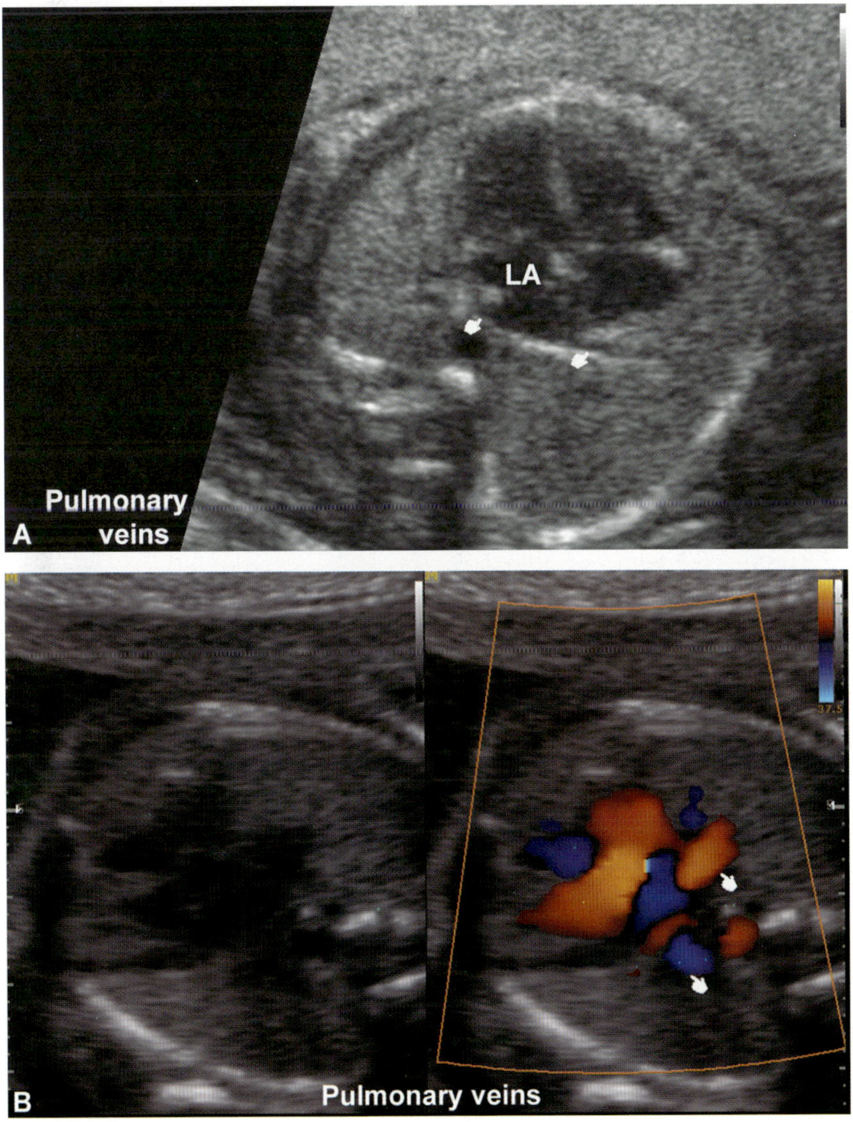

Figs 28A and B

LEFT ATRIUM

1. The left atrium is located posteriorly, near to the spine.
2. The left atrium receives the right and left pulmonary veins with a total of four pulmonary veins.
3. Routinely at the level of the four-chamber view, two of the four pulmonary veins are seen as slitlike openings in the posterior wall of the left atrium.
4. The left atrium also receives blood from the right atrium via the foramen ovale.
5. Blood flows through the left atrium to the left ventricle via the bicuspid (mitral) valve.

1. The left atrium (LA) is located posteriorly, near to the spine (Fig. 29).

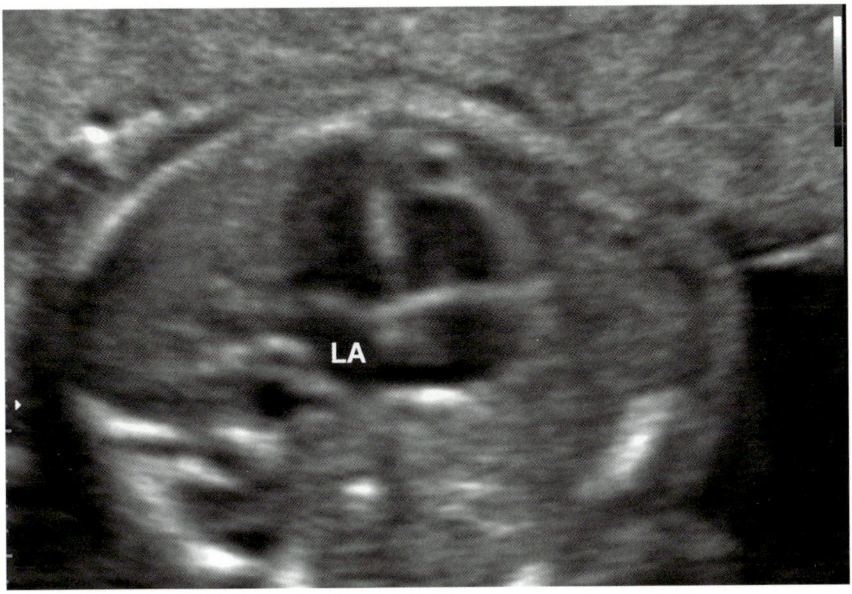

Fig. 29

2. The left atrium (LA) receives the right and left pulmonary veins with a total of four pulmonary veins (Fig. 30).

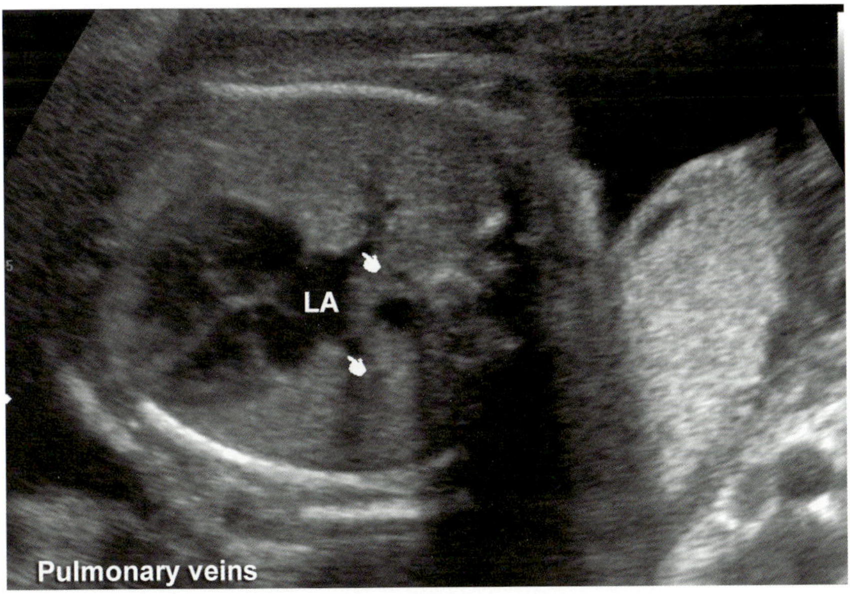

Fig. 30

3. Routinely at the level of the four-chamber view, two of the four pulmonary veins are seen as slitlike openings in the posterior wall of the left atrium (LA) (Fig. 31).

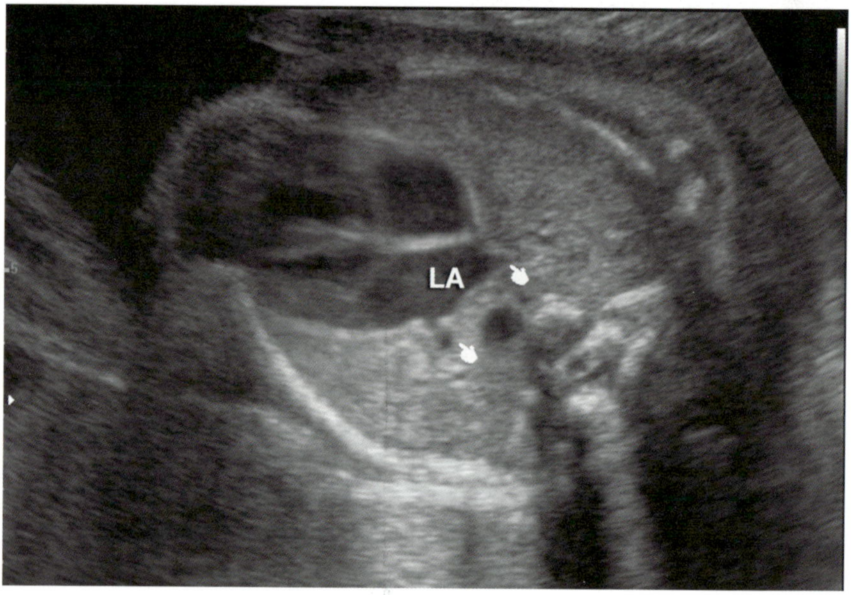

Fig. 31

4. The left atrium (LA) also receives blood from the right atrium (RA) via the foramen ovale (Figs 32A and B).

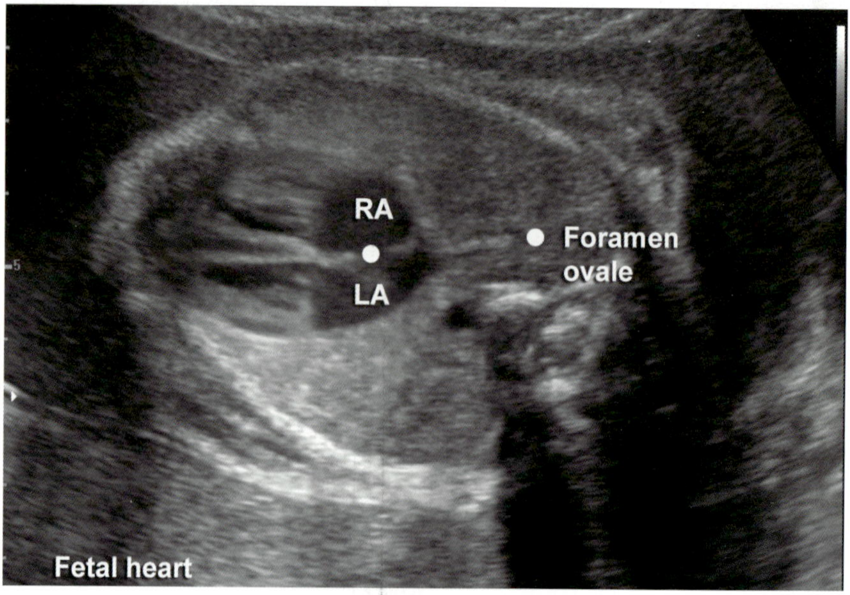

Fig. 32A

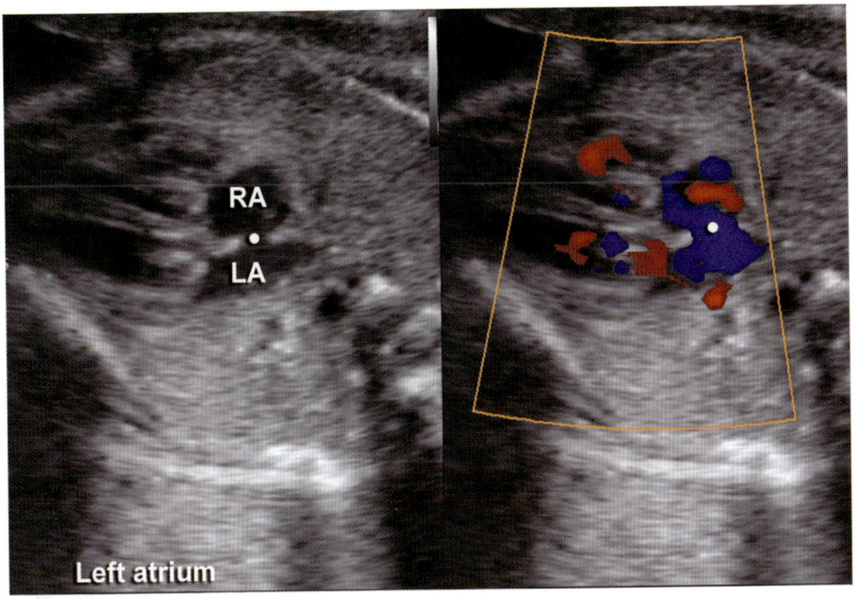

Fig. 32B

5. Blood flows through the left atrium (LA) to the left ventricle (LV) via the bicuspid (mitral) valve (Fig. 33).

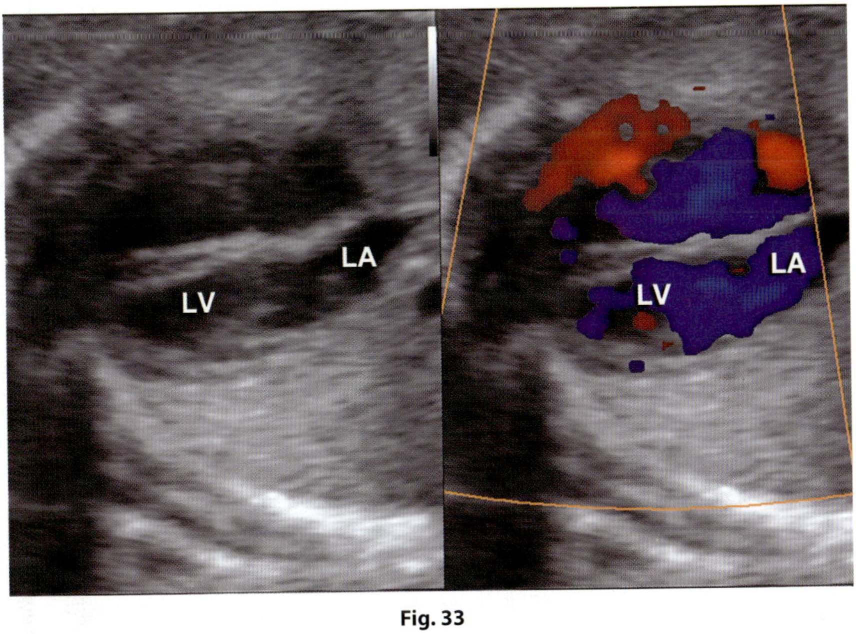

Fig. 33

MITRAL/BICUSPID VALVE

1. The mitral valve is located between the left atrium and left ventricle.
2. Blood flows from the left atrium to the left ventricle (one-way).
3. Mitral valve does not allow blood from flowing back into the left atrium from the left ventricle during ventricular systole.

1. The mitral valve is located between the left atrium (LA) and left ventricle (LV) (Figs 34A and B).

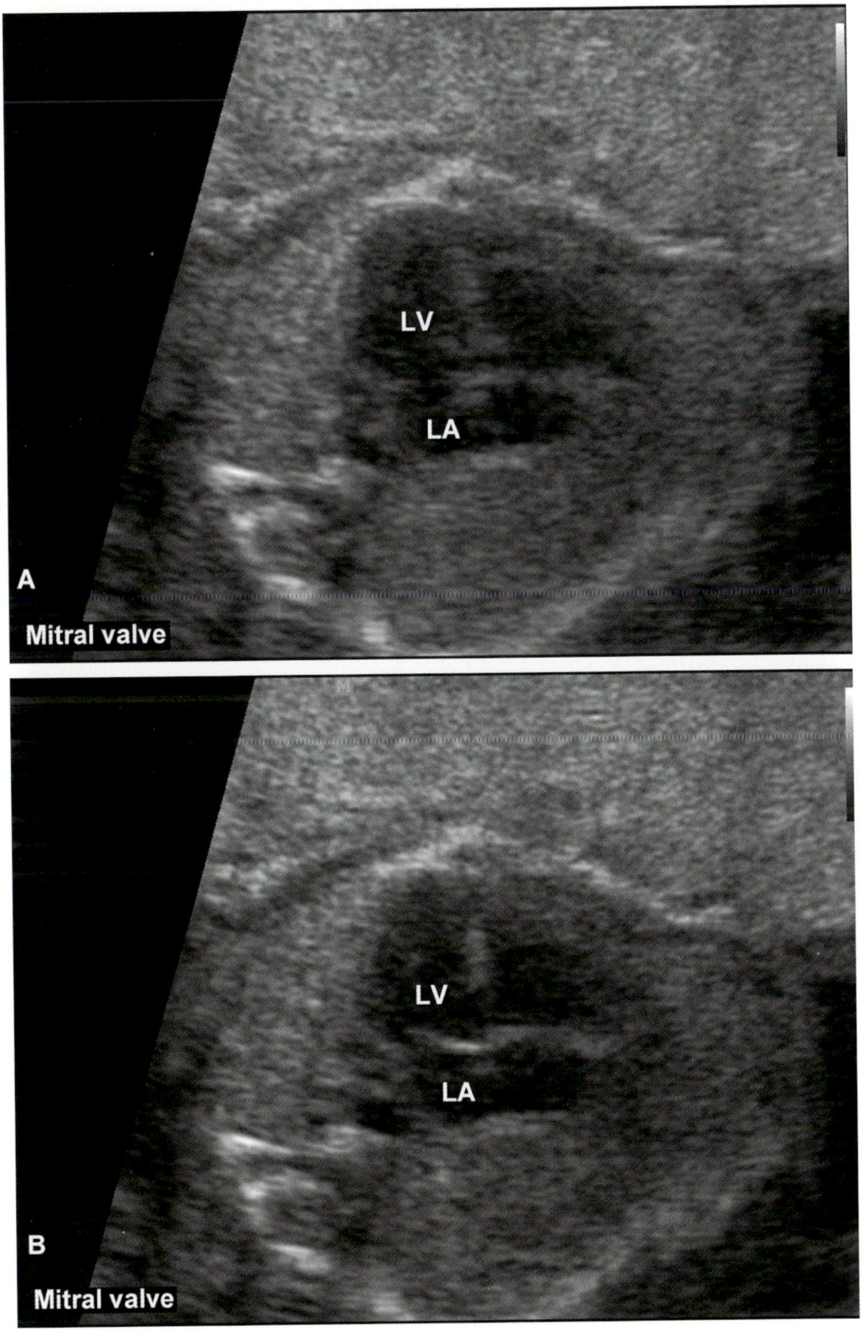

Figs 34A and B

2. Blood flows from the left atrium (LA) to the left ventricle (LV) (one-way) (Figs 35A and B).

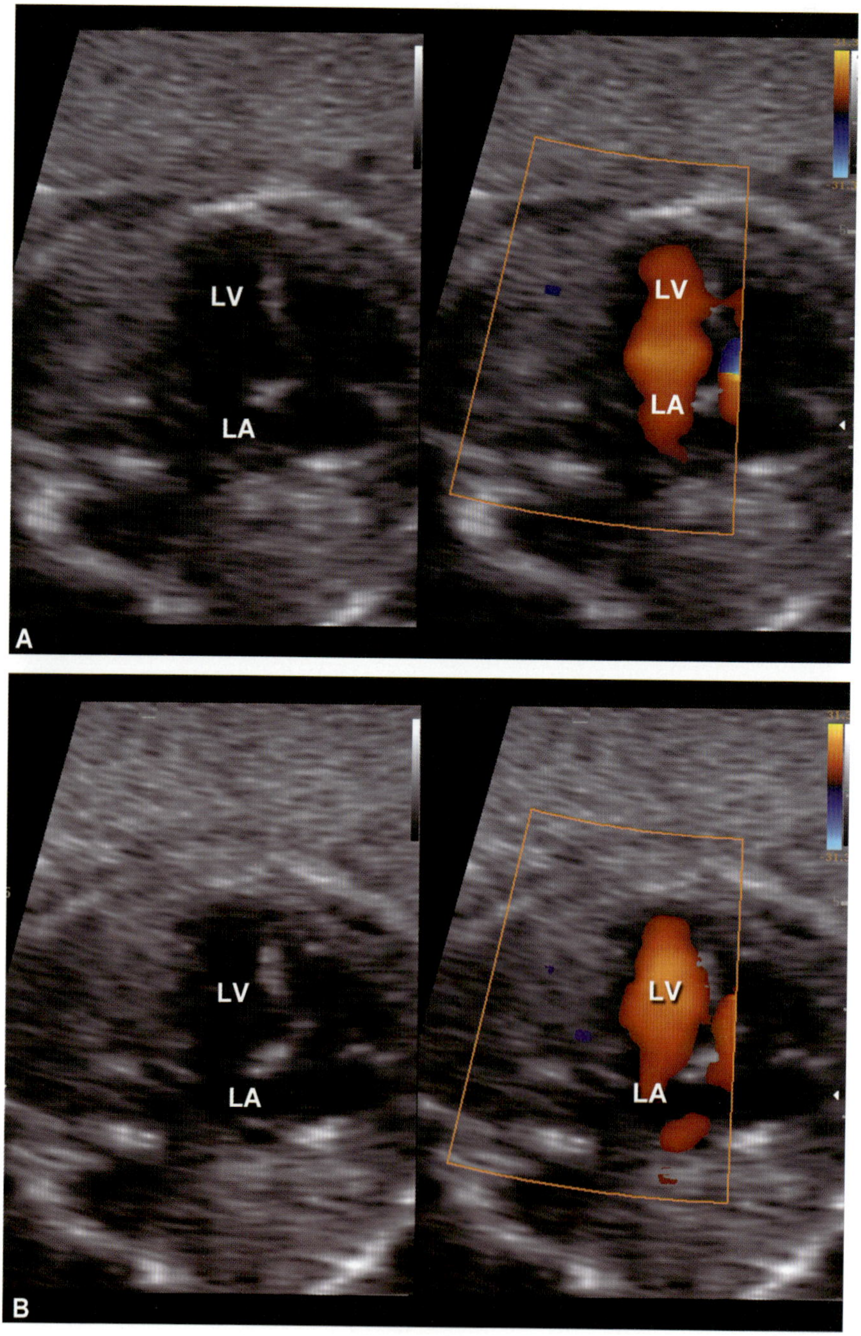

Figs 35A and B

3. Mitral valve does not allow blood from flowing back into the left atrium from the left ventricle during ventricular systole (Fig. 36).

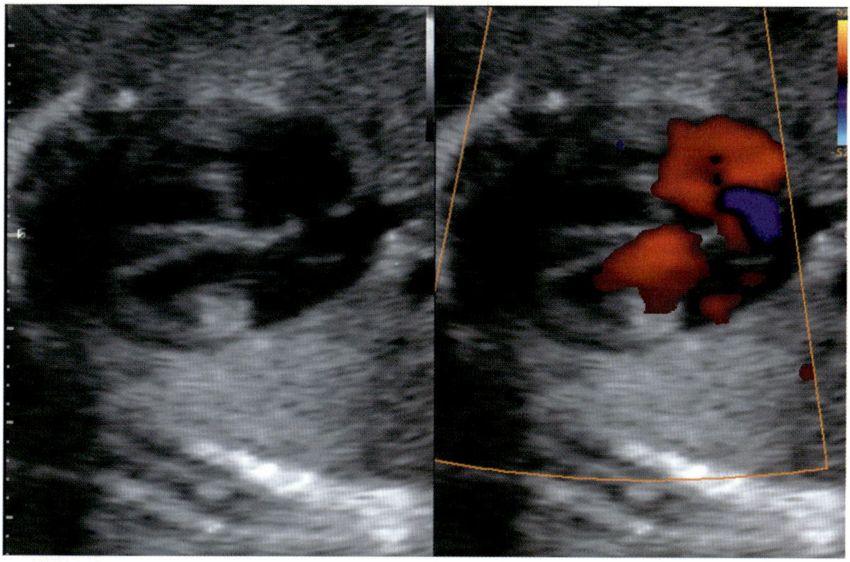

Fig. 36

LEFT VENTRICLE

1. The left ventricle is conical in shape and is located posterior to the right ventricle.
2. Most of the left lateral surface of the fetal heart is occupied by the left ventricle.
3. The inflow into the left ventricle is through the bicuspid valve/mitral valve.
4. The outflow tract of the left ventricle is the aorta.

1. The left ventricle (LV) is conical in shape and is located posterior to the right ventricle (Fig. 37).

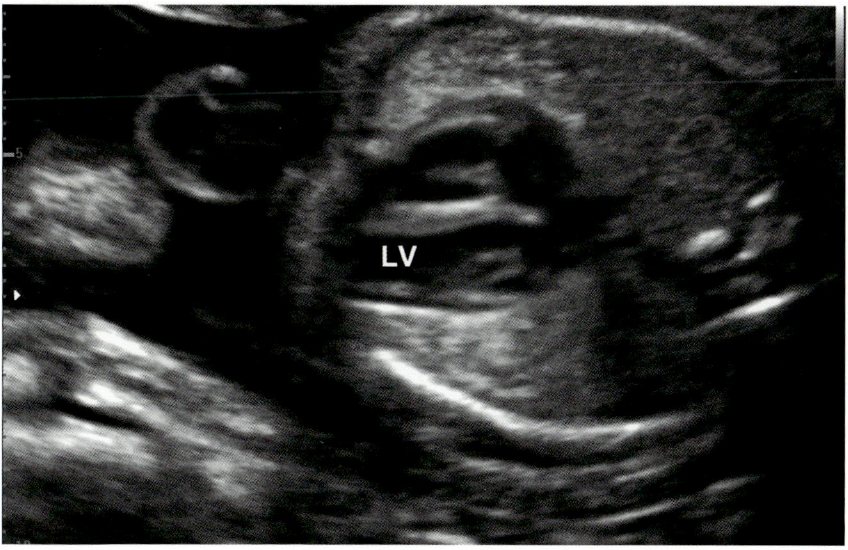

Fig. 37

2. Most of the left lateral surface of the fetal heart is occupied by the left ventricle (LV) (Fig. 38).

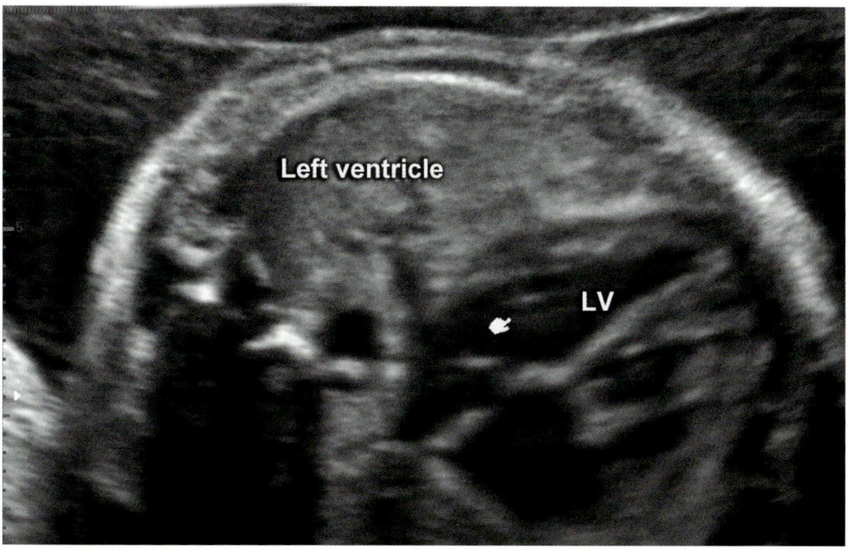

Fig. 38

3. The inflow into the left ventricle (LV) is through the bicuspid valve/mitral valve (Fig. 39).

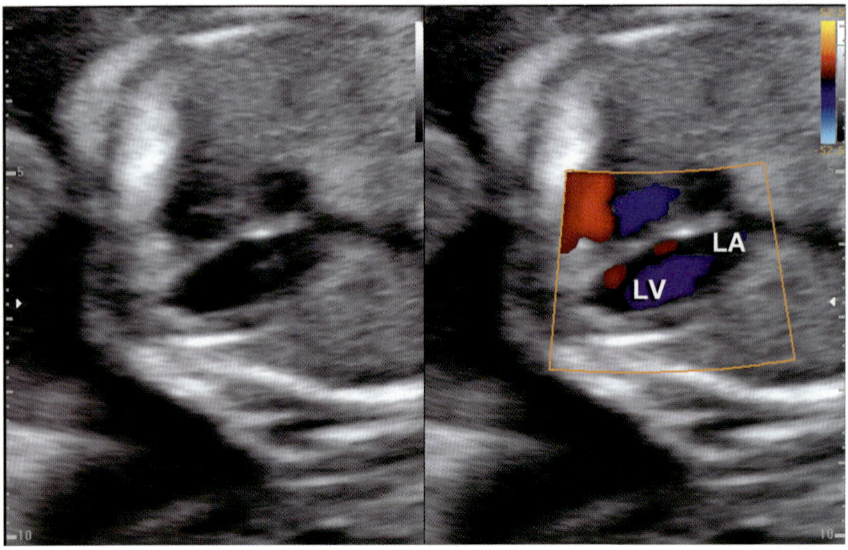

Fig. 39

4. The outflow tract of the left ventricle (LV) is the aorta (Ao) (Figs 40A and B).

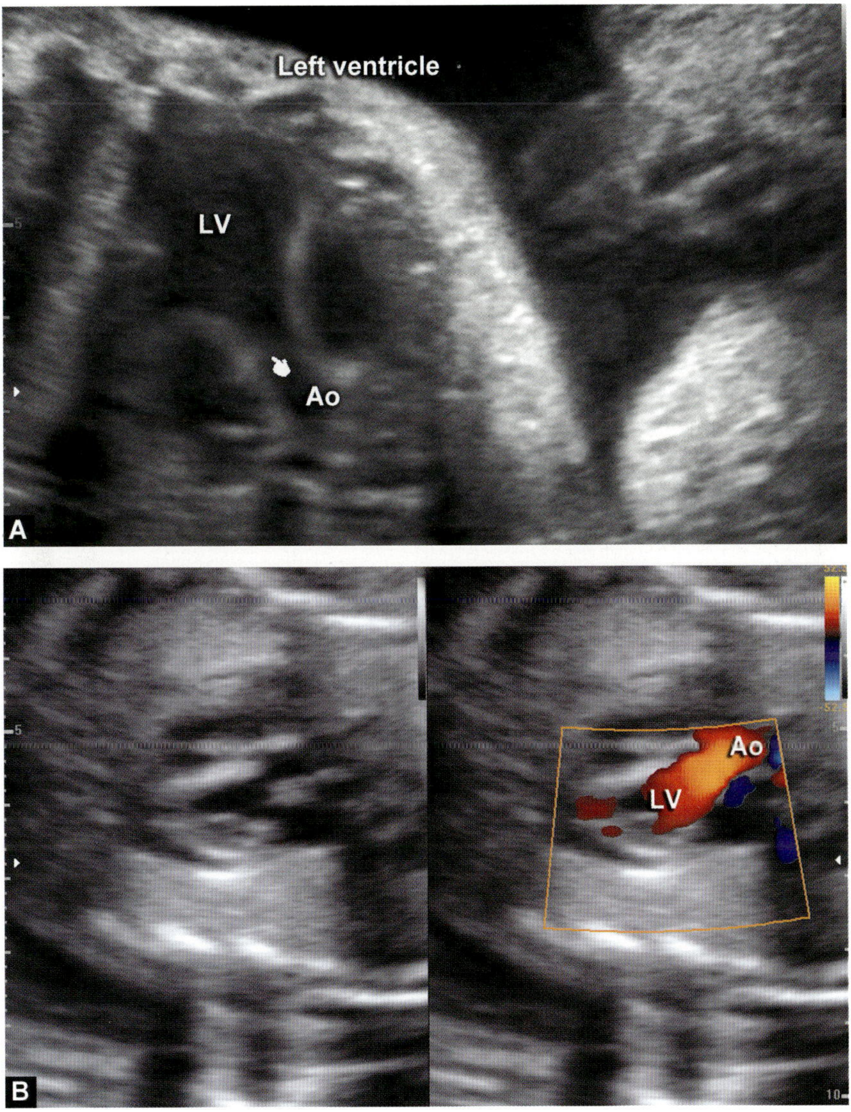

Figs 40A and B

AORTA

1. The ascending aorta arises from the left ventricle in the central portion of the heart.
2. It angles anteriorly, pointing towards the fetal right shoulder and parallel to the long-axis of the left ventricle.
3. The ascending aorta is bordered anteriorly by the interventricular septum and posteriorly by the anterior leaflet of the mitral valve.
4. The ascending aorta passes between the right and left atrium and inferior to the pulmonary artery before it emerges from the heart and curves posteriorly from the aortic arch.
5. The aortic arch gives rise to three arterial branches. Aortic arch branches distinguish the aortic arch from the ductal arch, which gives no branches as it connects with the descending aorta.
6. During left ventricular diastole, blood is prevented from flowing back into the ventricle by the aortic semilunar valve.

1. The ascending aorta (AAo) arises from the left ventricle (LV) in the central portion of the heart (Fig. 41).

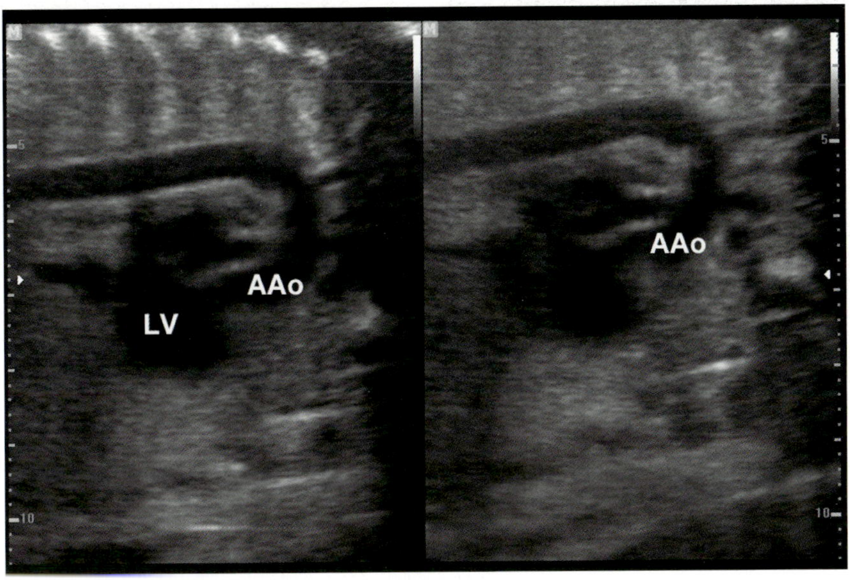

Fig. 41

2. It angles anteriorly, pointing towards the fetal right shoulder and parallel to the long-axis of the left ventricle (LV) (Fig. 42).

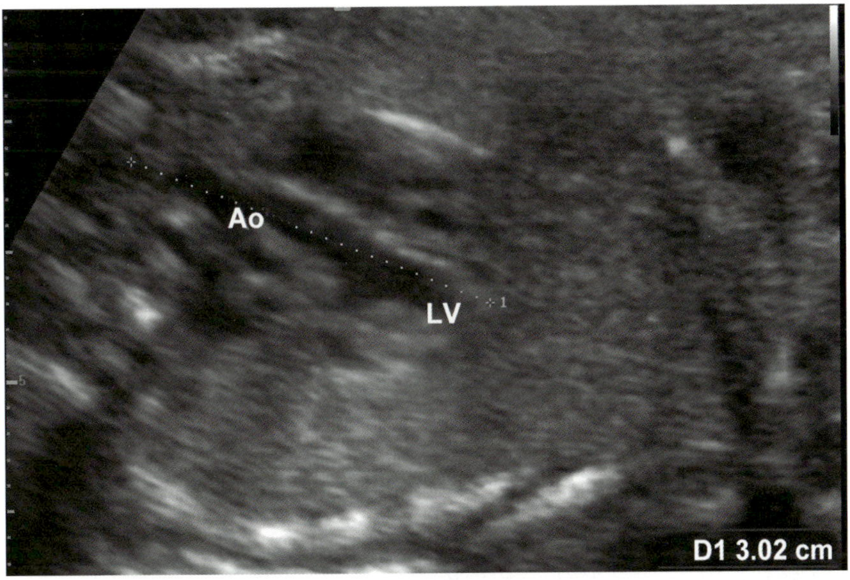

Fig. 42

3. The ascending aorta is bordered anteriorly by the interventricular septum and posteriorly by the anterior leaflet of the mitral valve (Fig. 43).

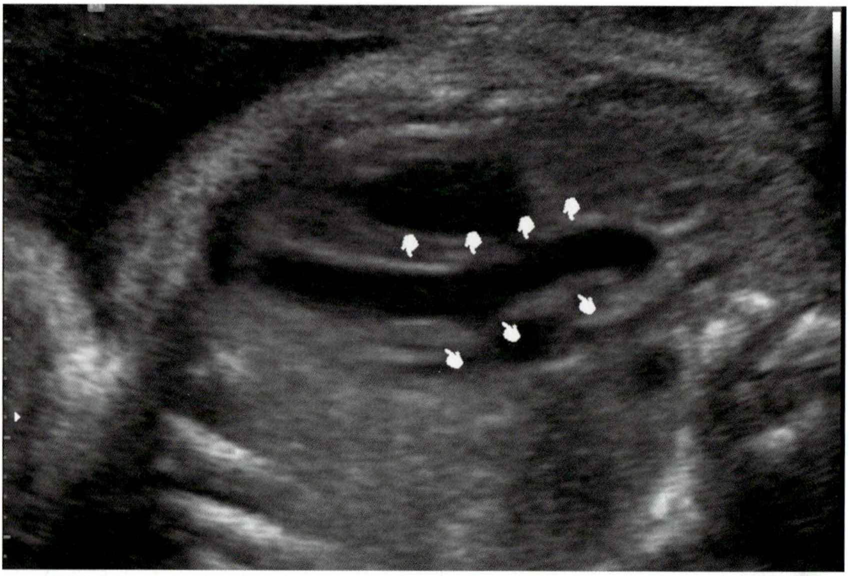

Fig. 43

4. The ascending aorta (Ao) passes between the right atrium (RA) and left atrium (LA) and inferior to the pulmonary artery before it emerges from the heart and curves posteriorly from the aortic arch (Fig. 44).

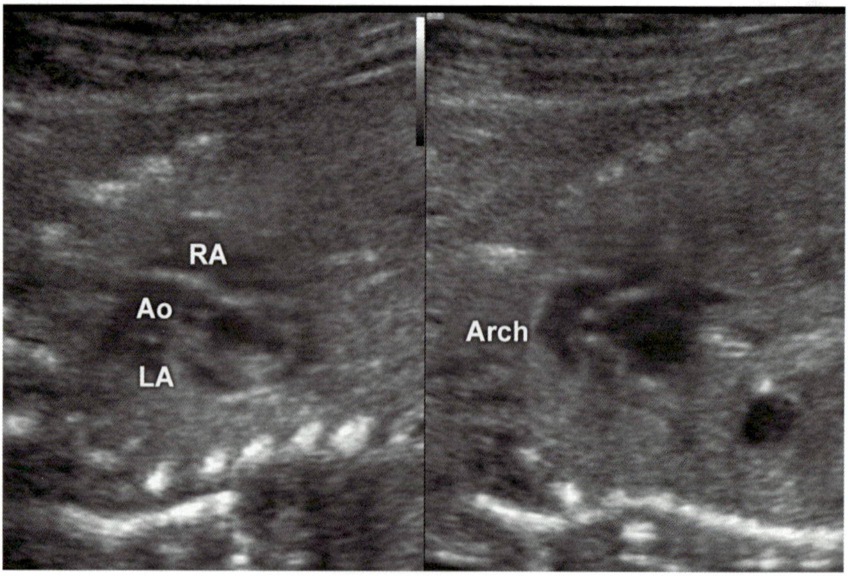

Fig. 44

5. The aortic arch gives rise to three arterial branches. Aortic arch branches distinguish the aortic arch from the ductal arch, which gives no branches as it connects with the descending aorta (Fig. 45).

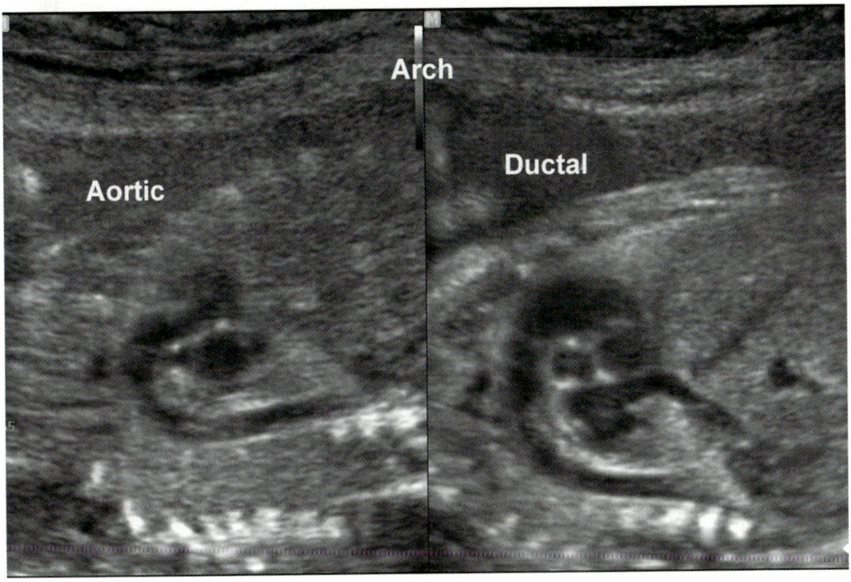

Fig. 45

6. During left ventricular diastole, blood is prevented from flowing back into the ventricle by the aortic semilunar valve (Fig. 46).

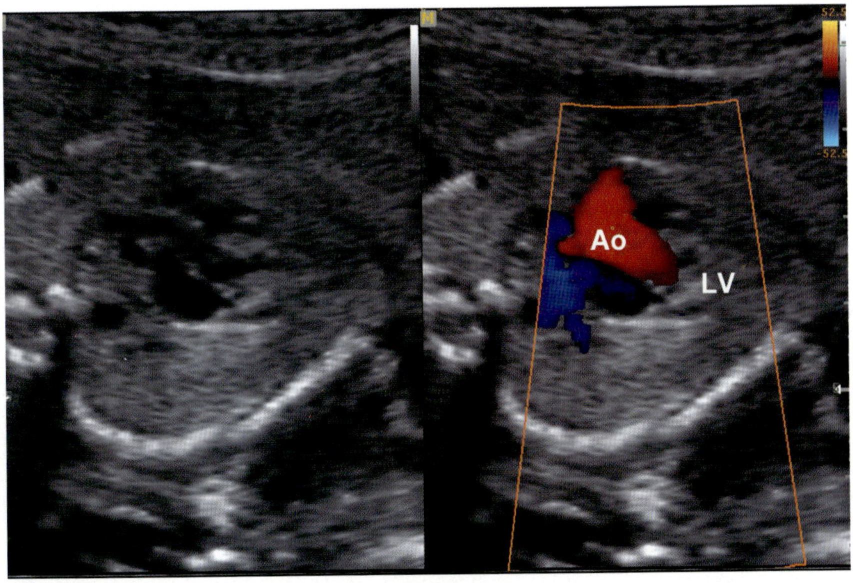

Fig. 46

FORAMEN OVALE

1. Foramen ovale occupies the middle third of the atrial septum.
2. The flap of the foramen ovale moves within the left atrial chamber as blood flows from the right atrium to the left atrium.
3. The foramen ovale may be imaged when the interatrial septum is parallel, tangential, or perpendicular to the septum.

1. Foramen ovale occupies the middle third of the atrial septum (Fig. 47).

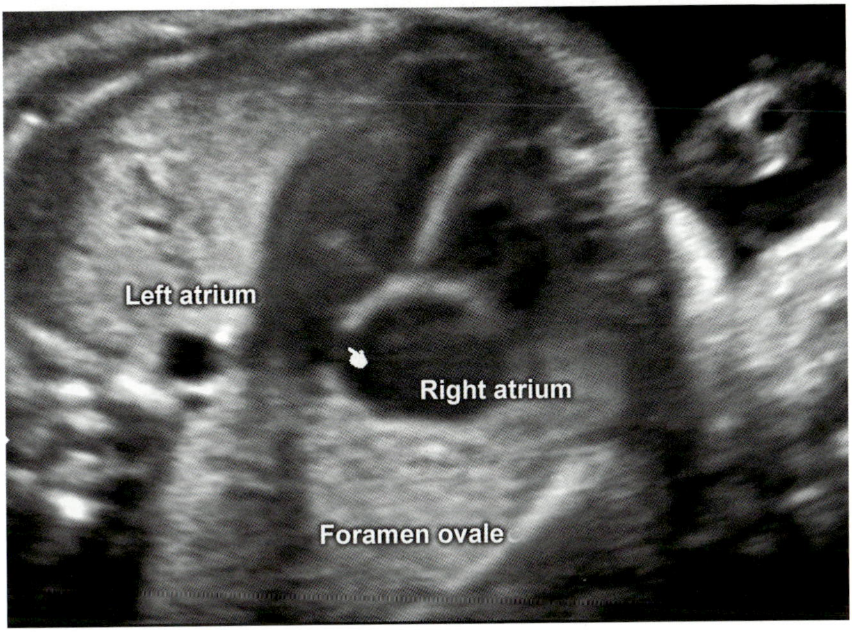

Fig. 47

2. The flap of the foramen ovale moves within the left atrial chamber as blood flows from the right atrium (RA) to the left atrium (LA) (Figs 48A and B).

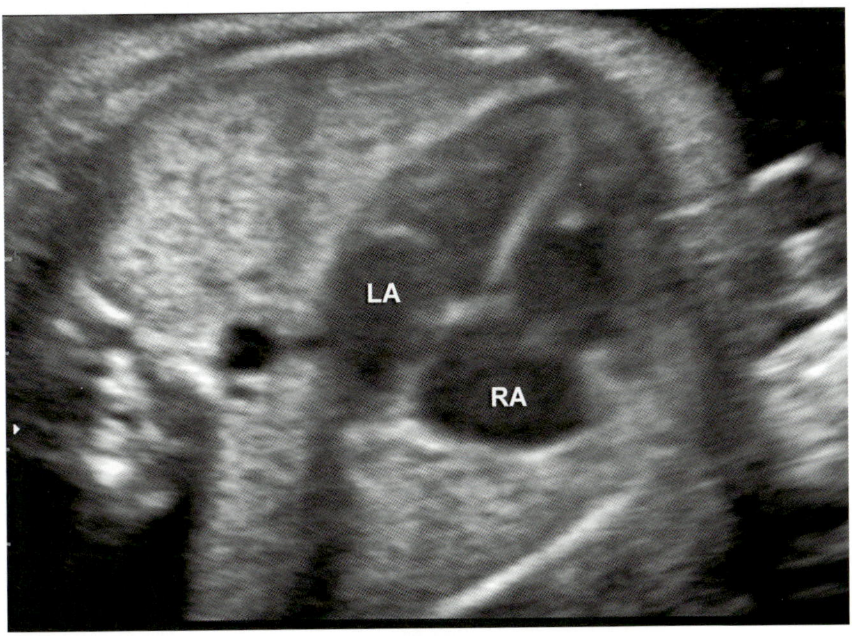

Fig. 48A

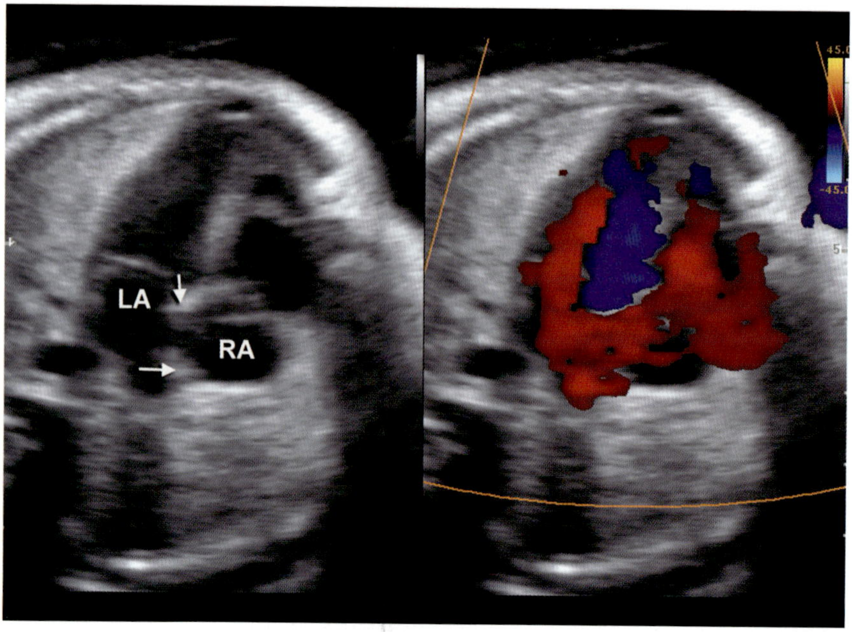

Fig. 48B

3. The foramen ovale may be imaged when the interatrial septum is parallel, tangential, or perpendicular to the septum (Fig. 49).

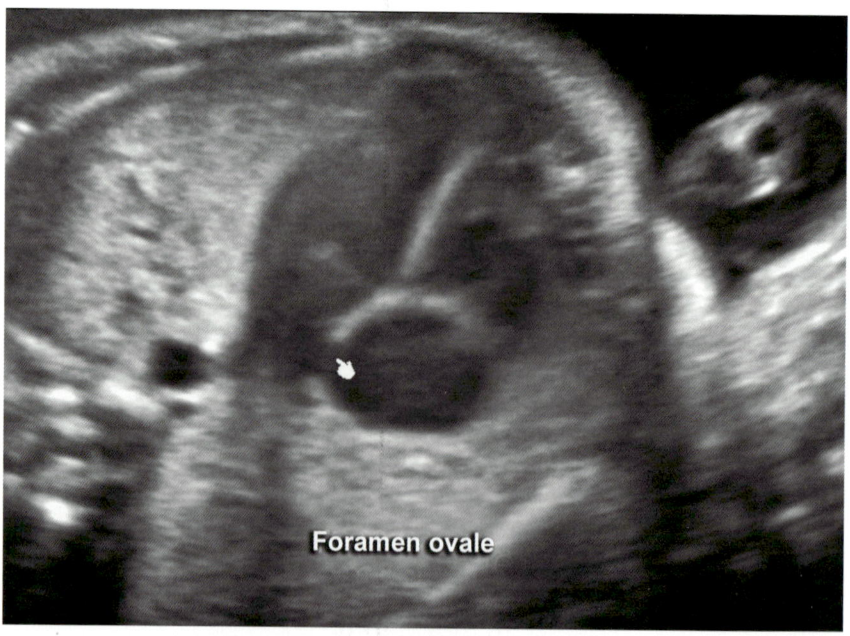

Fig. 49

INTERVENTRICULAR SEPTUM

1. The ventricles are separated by the ventricular septum.
2. The apical portion (nearer to the cardiac apex) is muscular in origin, and the basal portion (nearer to the atrioventricular valves) is membranous.
3. The ventricular septum ensures no mixing of blood between the two ventricles.

1. The ventricles are separated by the ventricular septum (Fig. 50).

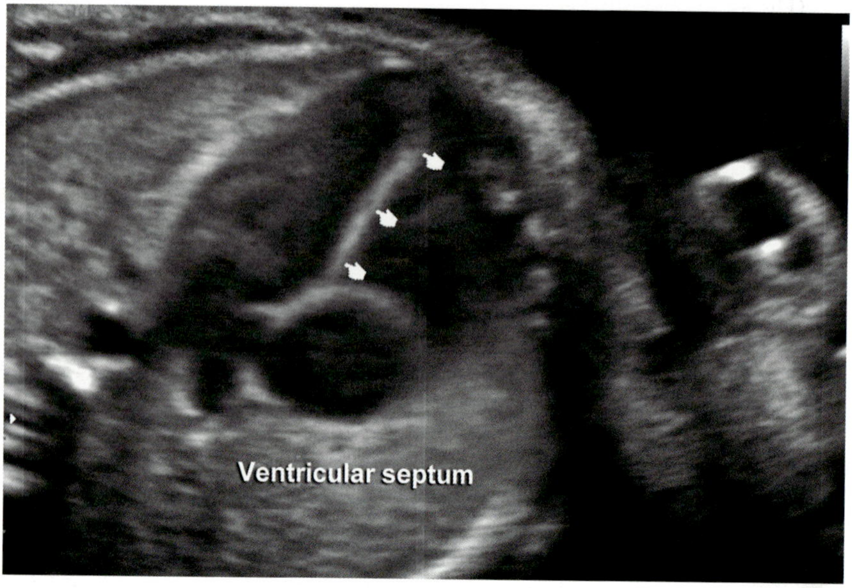

Fig. 50

2. The apical portion (nearer to the cardiac apex) is muscular in origin, and the basal portion (nearer to the atrioventricular valves) is membranous (Fig. 51).

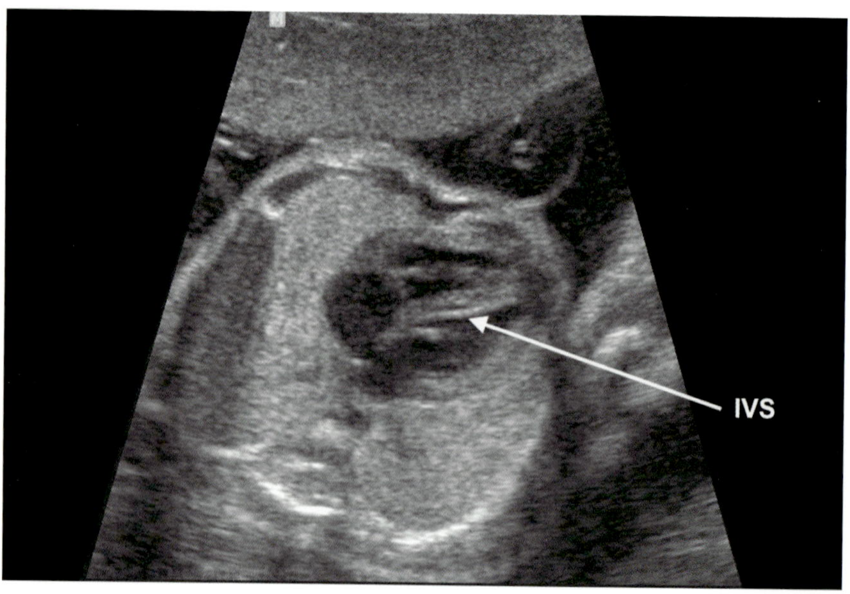

Fig. 51

3. The ventricular septum ensures no mixing of blood between the two ventricles (Fig. 52).

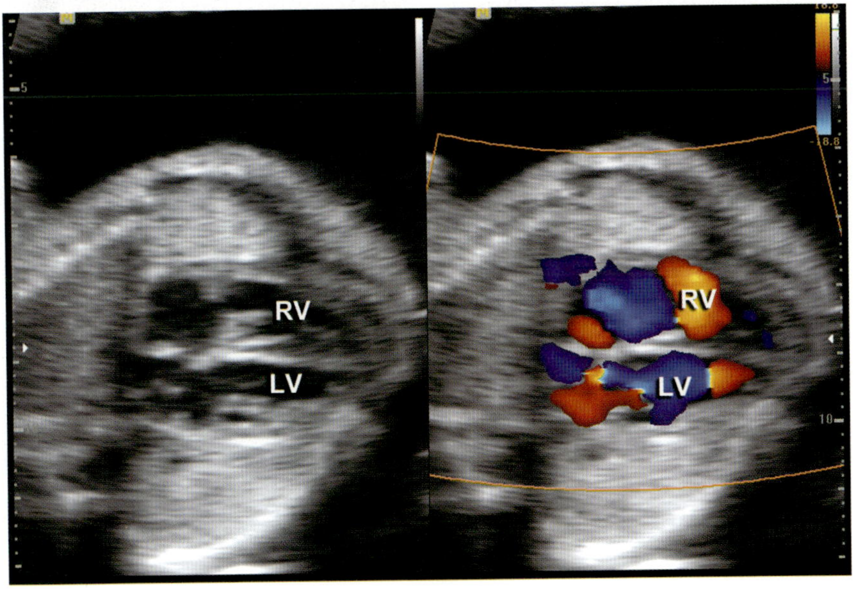

Fig. 52

8

Views

A. Transverse
   i. Cardiac Four-chamber View
   ii. Five-chamber View
   iii. Three Vessel View
   iv. Transverse Arterial Duct View
   v. Aortic Arch Transverse View
   vi. Three-Vessel Trachea View

B. Sagittal
   i. Bicaval View
   ii. Aortic Arch View
   iii. Ductal Arch View

C. Oblique
   i. Right Ventricular Outflow View
   ii. Left Ventricular Long-axis View
   iii. Ventricular Short-axis View

TRANSVERSE

Four-chamber View

1. Ascertain the fetal situs with fetal stomach, cardiac apex, position of aorta and IVC.
2. Transverse section of the fetal abdomen showing the fetal stomach and one rib laterally is the perfect plane.
3. From the transverse plane of abdomen slide your transducer towards the fetal chest and stop till you get a perfect four-chamber view with visualization of the cardiac apex and base.
4. You can get three types of cardiac four-chamber views:
   a. Apical four-chamber view.
   b. Basal four-chamber view.
   c. Axial/lateral four-chamber view.
5. A normal four-chamber view should comprise of
   a. Two atrial chambers of same size.
   b. Two ventricular chambers of same size. To correctly evaluate whether the chambers are of equal size image, the four-chamber view perpendicular to interventricular septum.
   c. Two atrioventricular valves (mitral and tricuspid valves) of same size. Orient the interventricular septum parallel or tangential beam to get the best view.
   d. The atrial and ventricular septa join at the junction where the leaflets of both the atrioventricular valves insert into the ventricular septum. This is named as the crux of the heart. The right atrioventricular/tricuspid valve inserts lower than the left atrioventricular/bicuspid valve.
   e. The interventricular septum should be complete. Examine the septum parallel or tangential to the ultrasound beam to check it optimally.
   f. The interatrial septum should have a foramen ovale.
   g. Paired superior and inferior pulmonary veins are identified entering the left atrium.

1. Ascertain the fetal situs with fetal stomach, cardiac apex, position of aorta and IVC (Fig. 1).

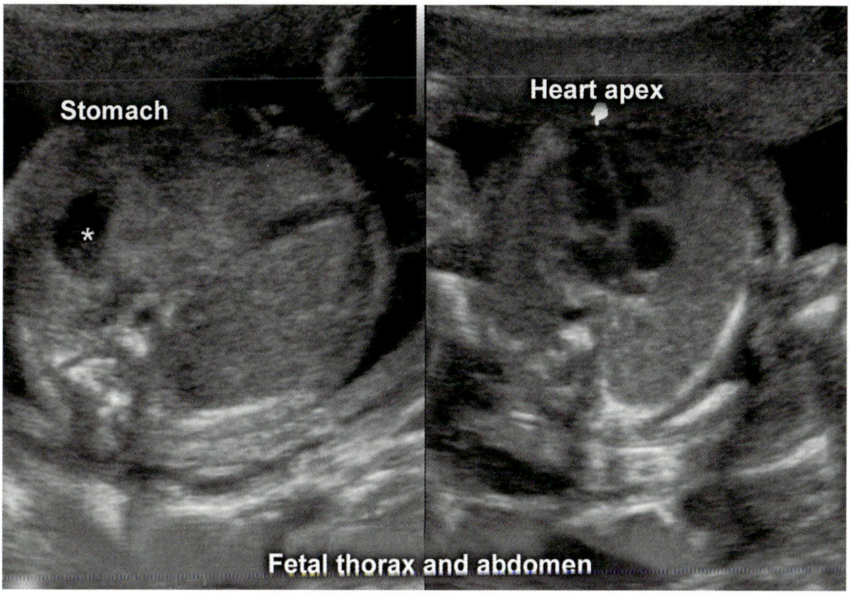

Fig. 1

2. Transverse section of the fetal abdomen showing the fetal stomach and one rib laterally is the perfect plane (Figs 2A and B).

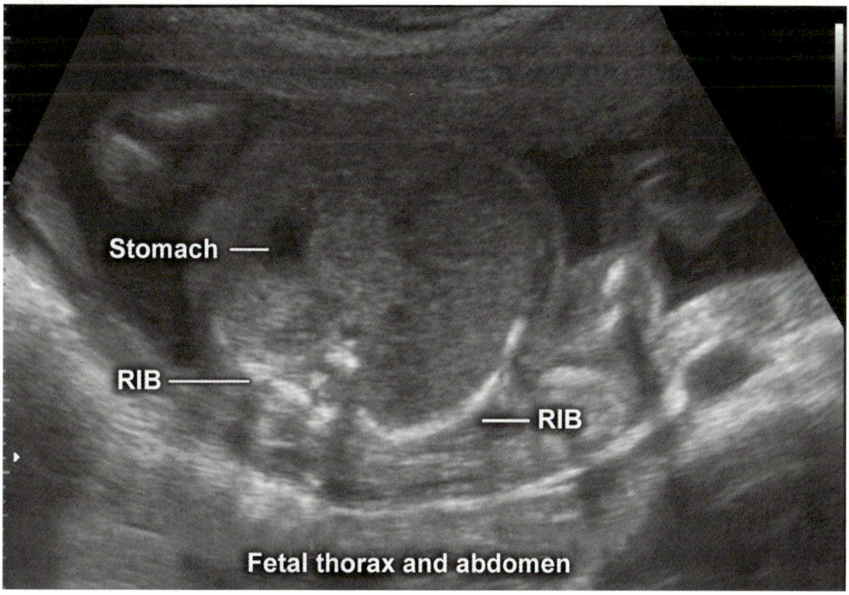

Fig. 2A

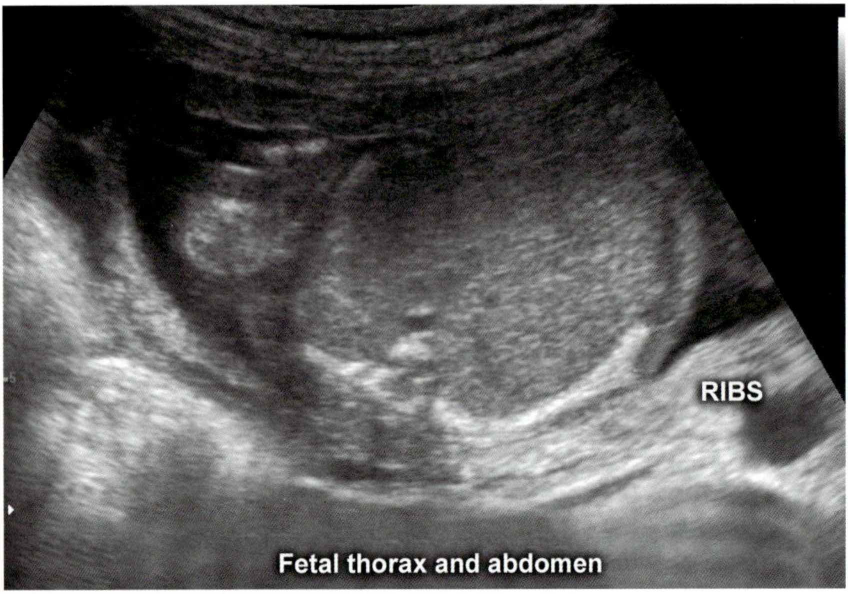

Fig. 2B

3. From the transverse plane of abdomen slide your transducer towards the fetal chest and stop till you get a perfect four-chamber view with visualization of the cardiac apex and base (Fig. 3).

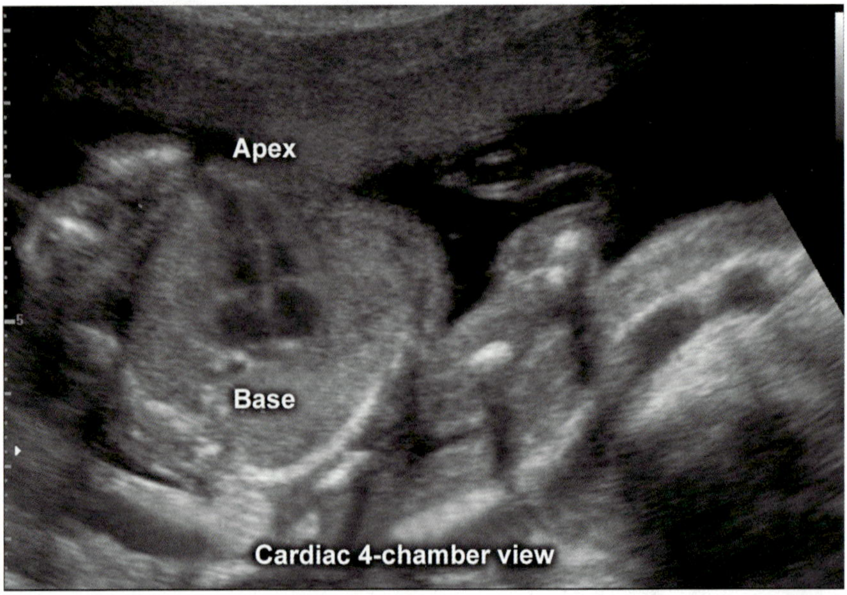

Fig. 3

4. You can get three types of cardiac four-chamber views.
   a. Apical four-chamber view (Fig. 4A).
   b. Basal four-chamber view (Fig. 4B).
   c. Axial/lateral four-chamber view (Fig. 4C).

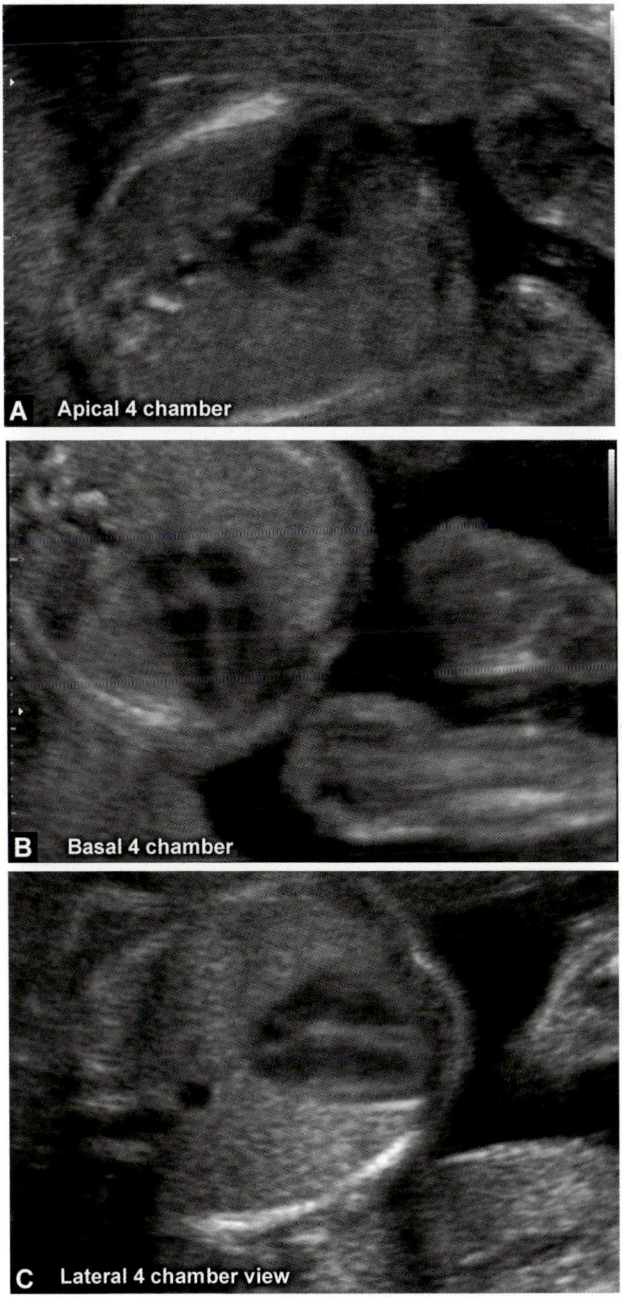

Figs 4A to C

5. A normal four-chamber view should comprise of:
   a. Two atrial chambers of same size (Figs 5A and B).

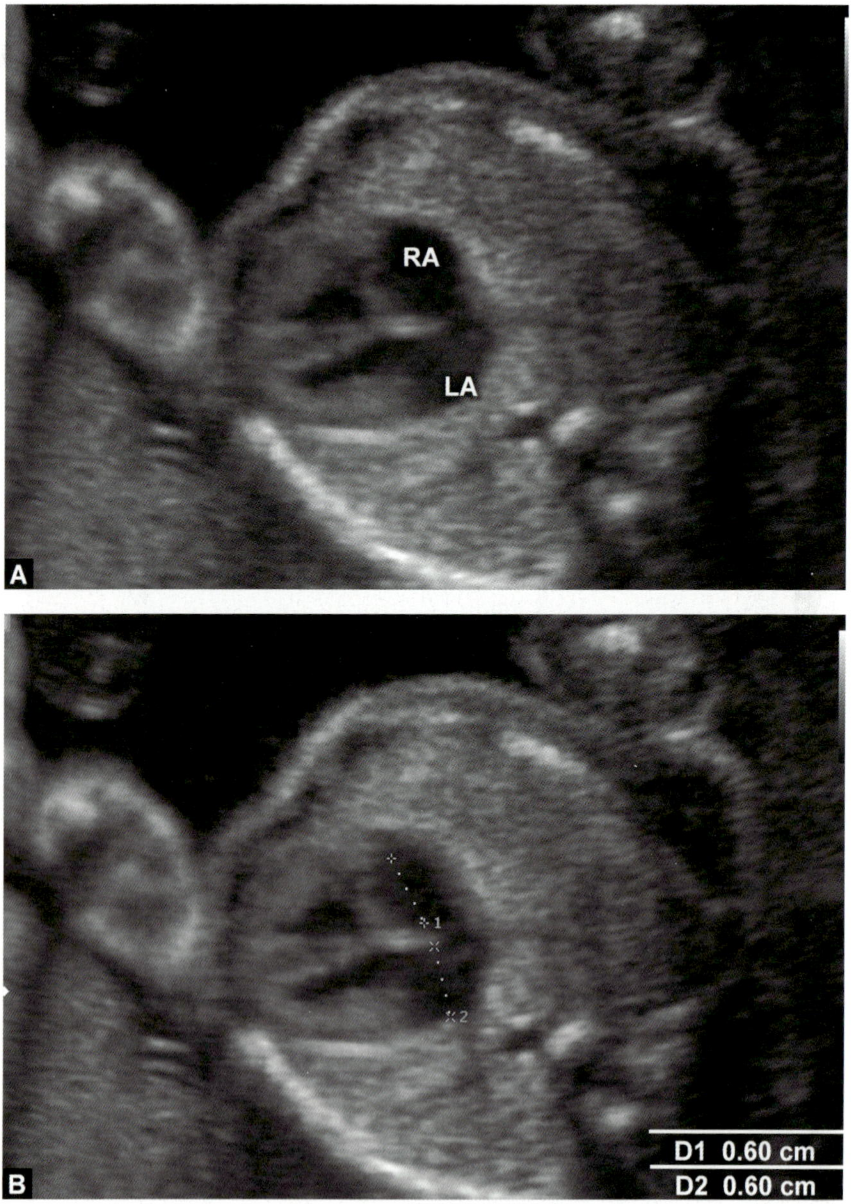

Figs 5A and B

b. Two ventricular chambers of same size. To correctly evaluate whether the chambers are of equal size image, the four-chamber view perpendicular to interventricular septum (Figs 6A and B).

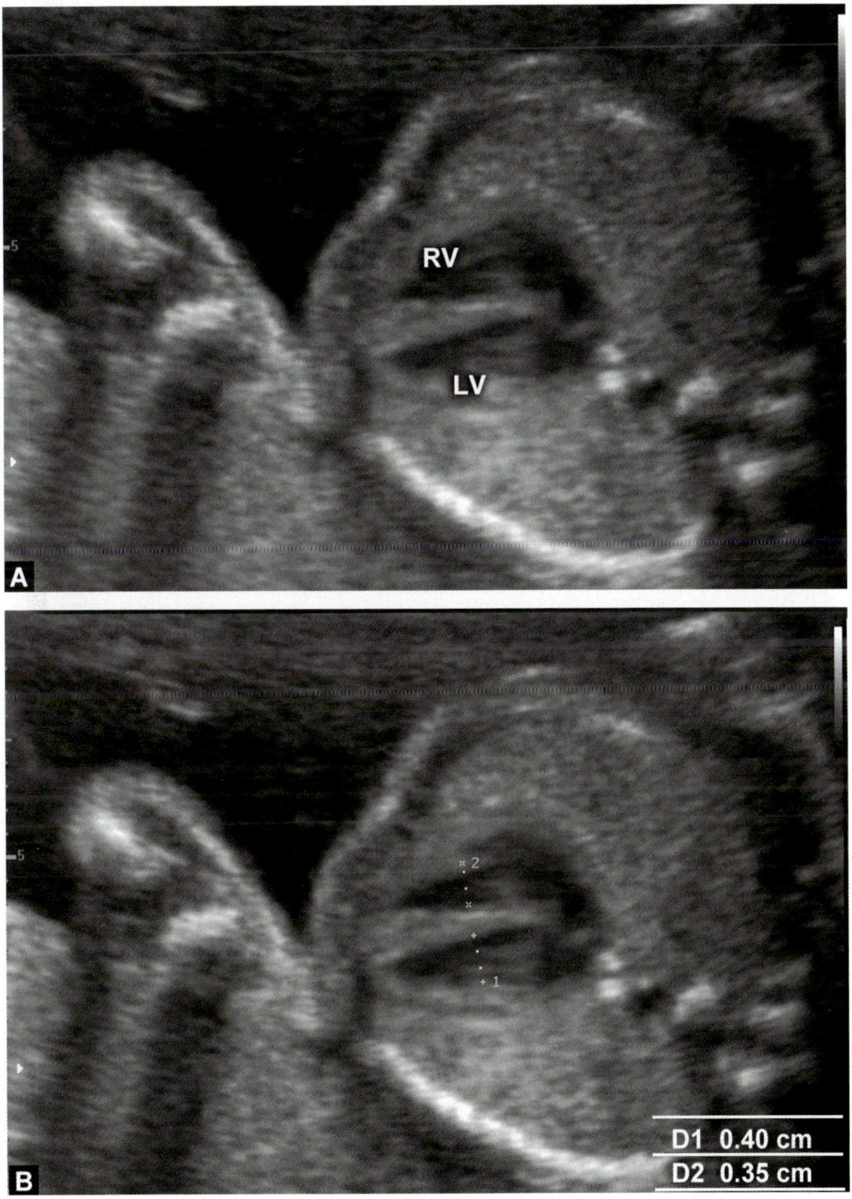

Figs 6A and B

c. Two atrioventricular valves (mitral and tricuspid valves) of same size. Orient the interventricular septum parallel or tangential beam to get the best view (Figs 7A and B).

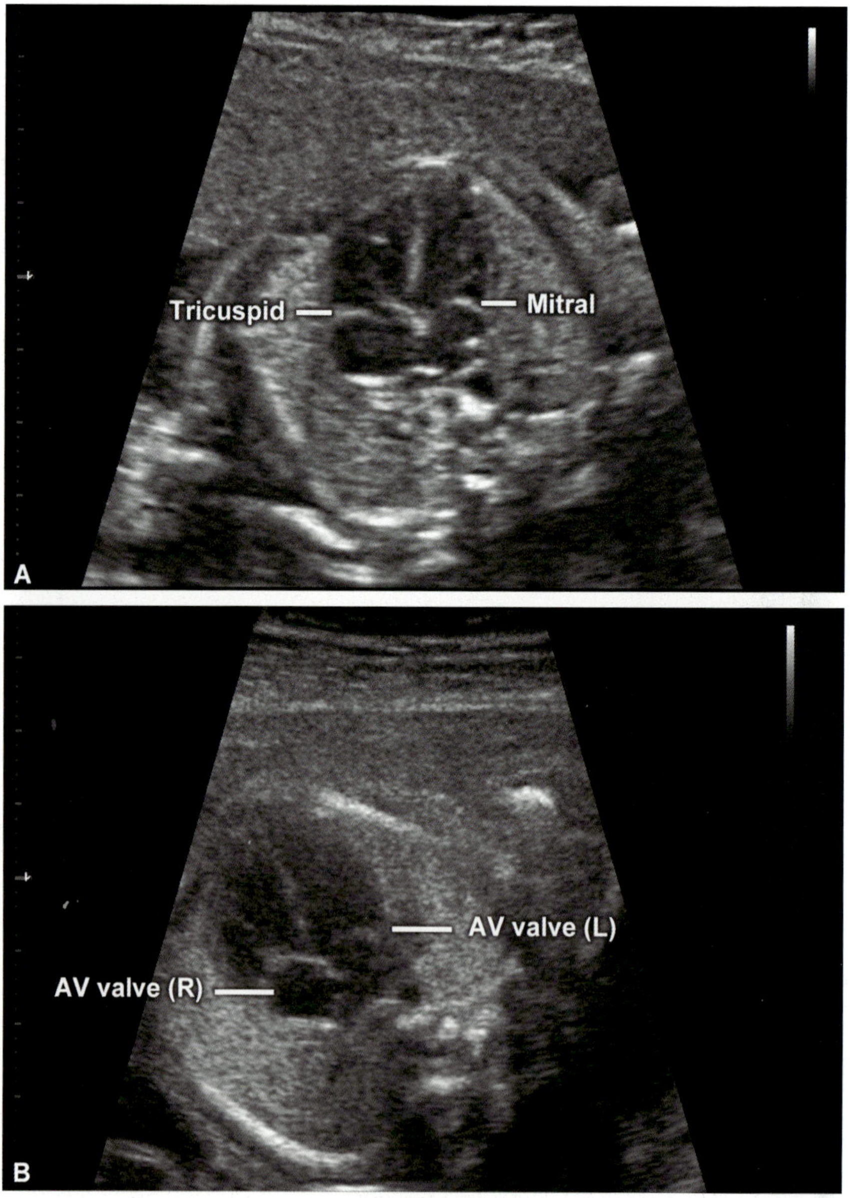

Figs 7A and B

d. The atrial and ventricular septa join at the junction where the leaflets of both the atrioventricular valves insert into the ventricular septum. This is named as the crux of the heart. The right atrioventricular/tricuspid valve inserts lower than the left atrioventricular/bicuspid valve (Figs 8A and B).

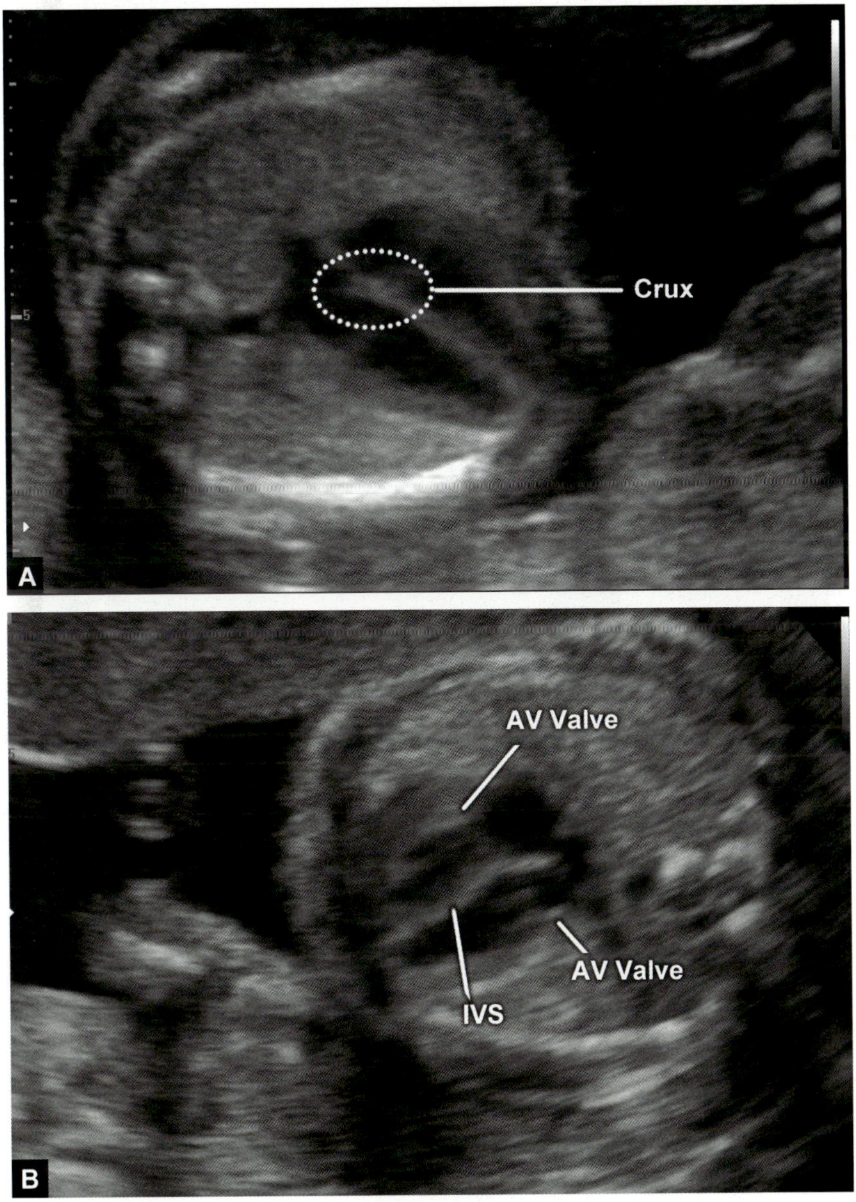

Figs 8A and B

e. The interventricular septum should be complete. Examine the septum parallel or tangential to the ultrasound beam to check it optimally (Figs 9A to C).

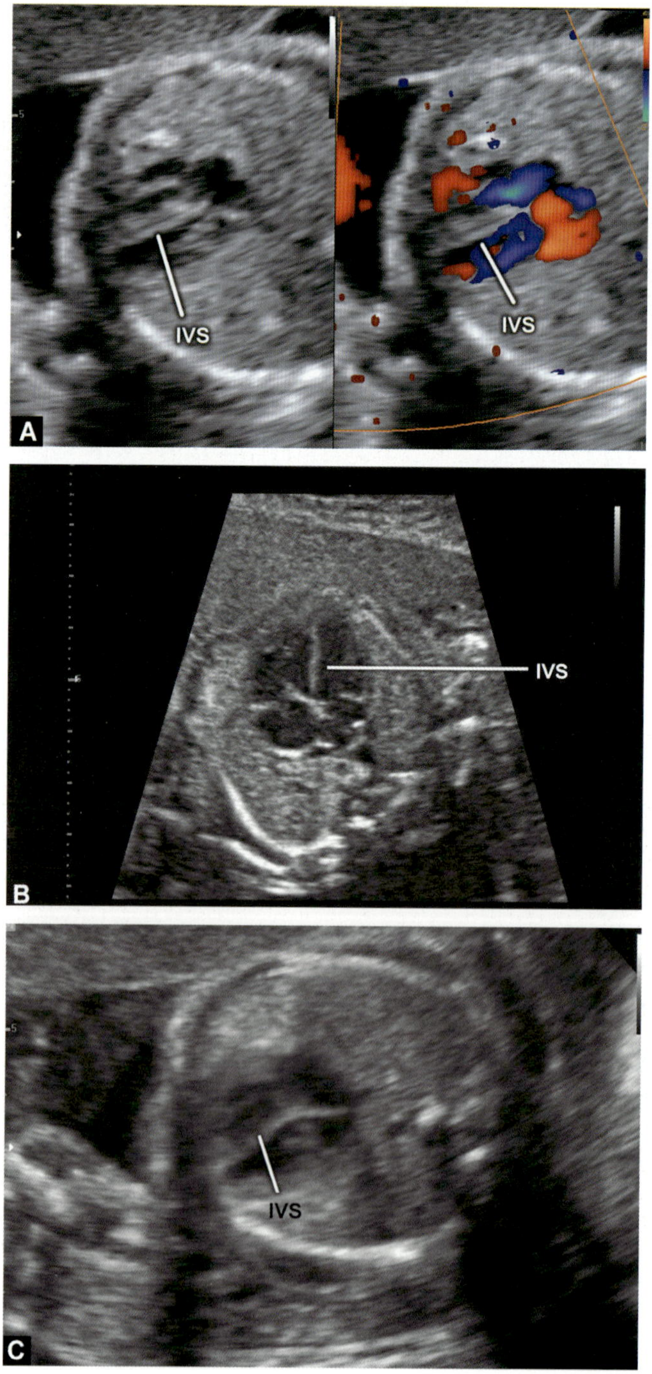

Figs 9A to C

f. The interatrial septum should have a foramen ovale (Fig. 10).

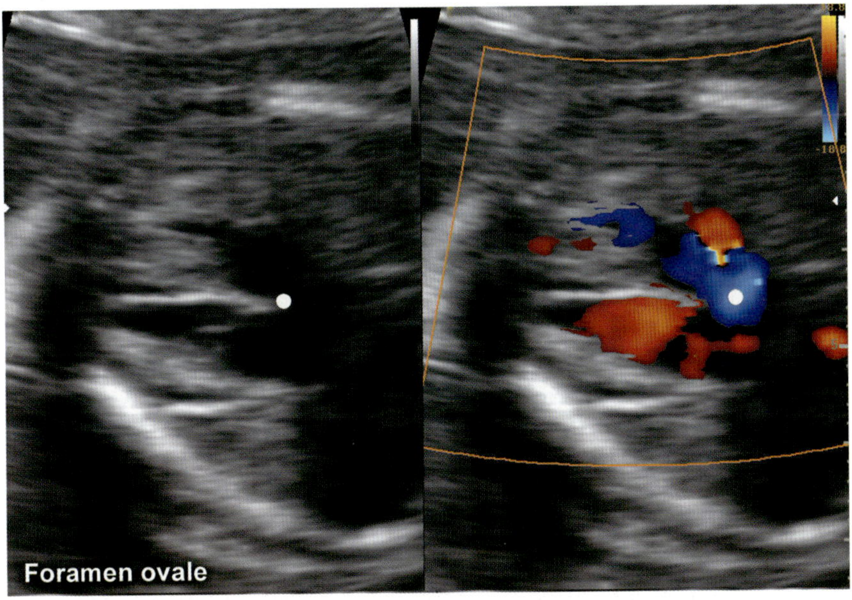

Fig. 10

g. Paired superior and inferior pulmonary veins are identified entering the left atrium (Fig. 11).

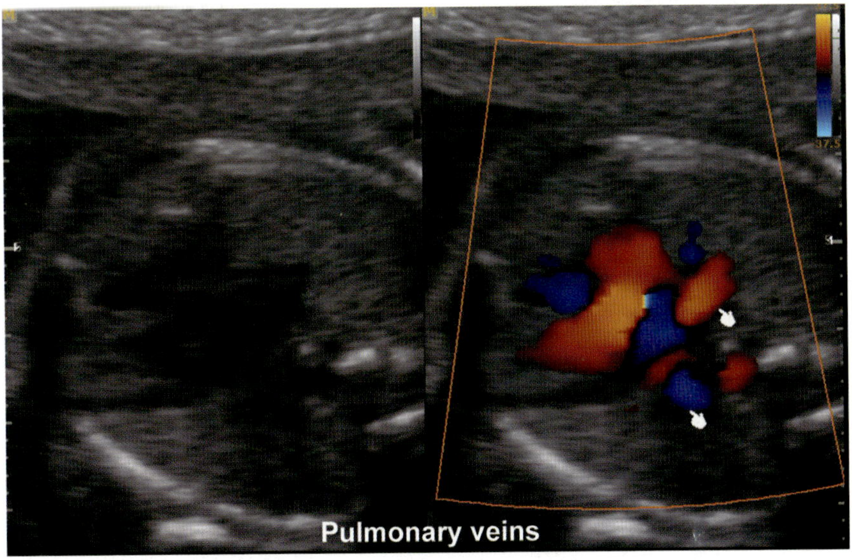

Fig. 11

Five-chamber View

1. The five-chamber view is a transverse plane which is obtained cephalad to the four-chamber view with a slight tilting towards the fetal head in order to get the ascending aorta in view.
2. In this view, the aortic route is seen in the center along with two ventricles and two atria. The two atrioventricular valves are seen on either side of the aorta.
3. The ascending aorta is the fifth component of the five-chamber view.
4. The ventricular septum and the anterior wall of the ascending aorta make a wide angle and should not appear in a straight line.
5. The ascending aorta forms the transverse aortic arch after it traverses between the two atria.
6. The superior wall of the ascending aorta is continuous with the interventricular septum.
7. The posterior wall of the aorta is continuous with the left atrioventricular valve.
8. All four chambers, the mitral valve and aorta are seen in this view. The tricuspid is not seen in the five-chamber view.

1. The five-chamber view is a transverse plane which is obtained cephalad to the four-chamber view with a slight tilting towards the fetal head in order to get the ascending aorta in view (Fig. 12).

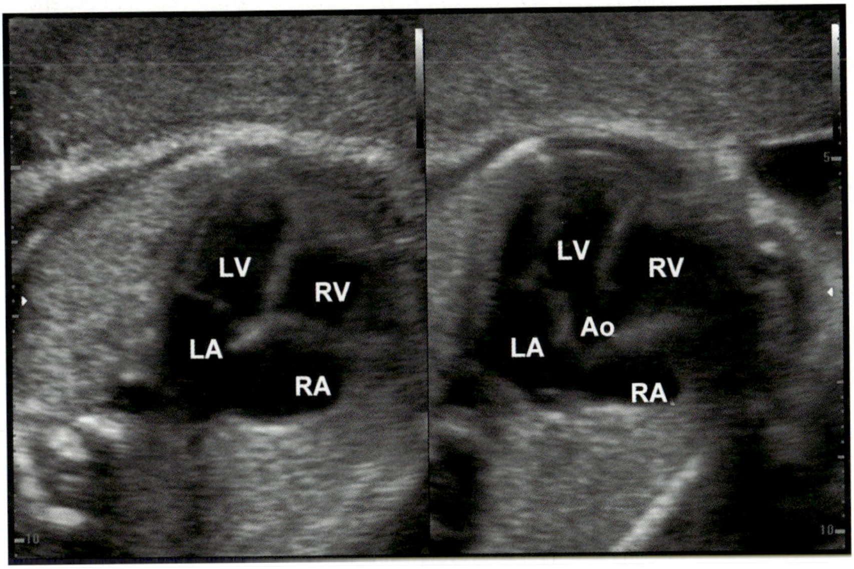

Fig. 12

2. In this view, the aortic route is seen in the center along with two ventricles and two atria. The two atrioventricular valves are seen on either side of the aorta (Fig. 13).

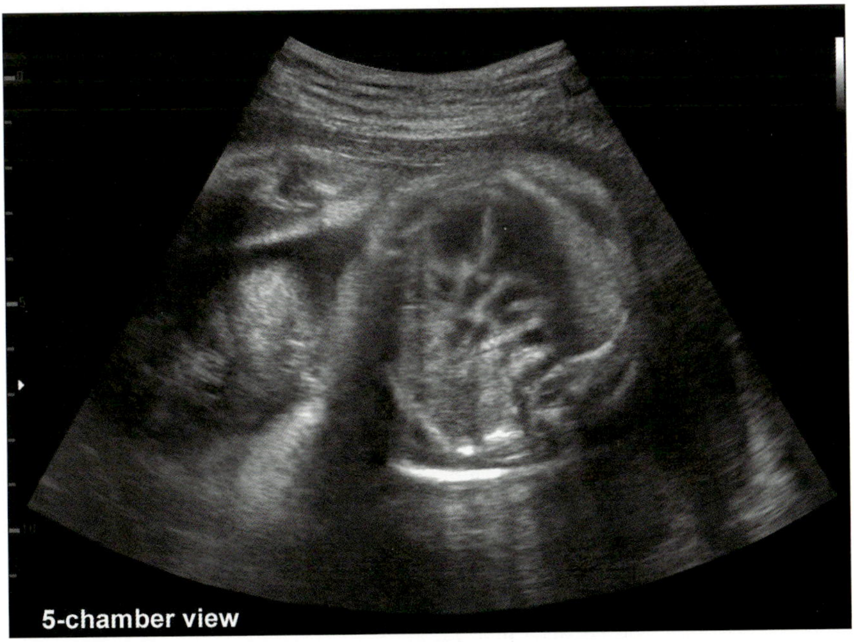

Fig. 13

3. The ascending aorta is the 5th component of the five-chamber view (Fig. 14).

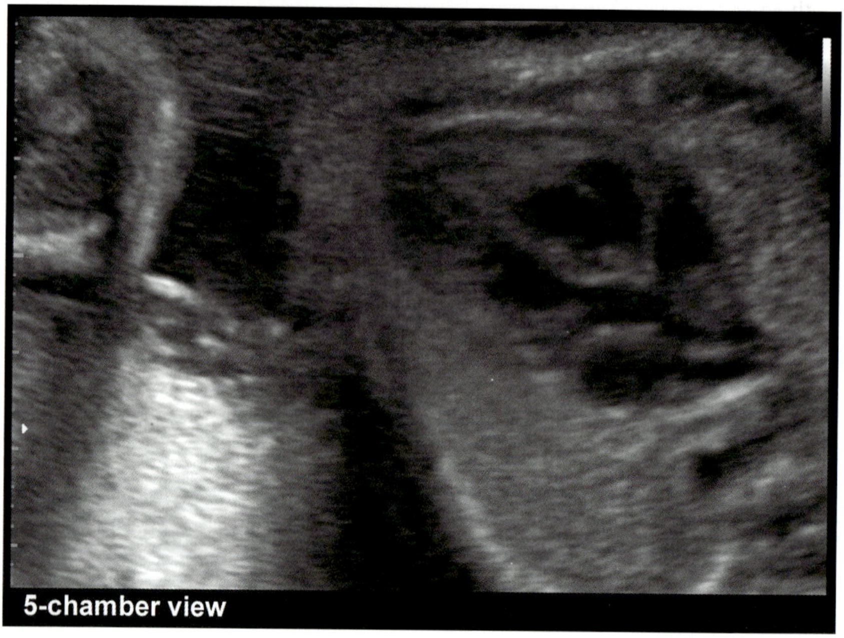

Fig. 14

4. The ventricular septum and the anterior wall of the ascending aorta make a wide angle and should not appear in a straight line (Fig. 15).

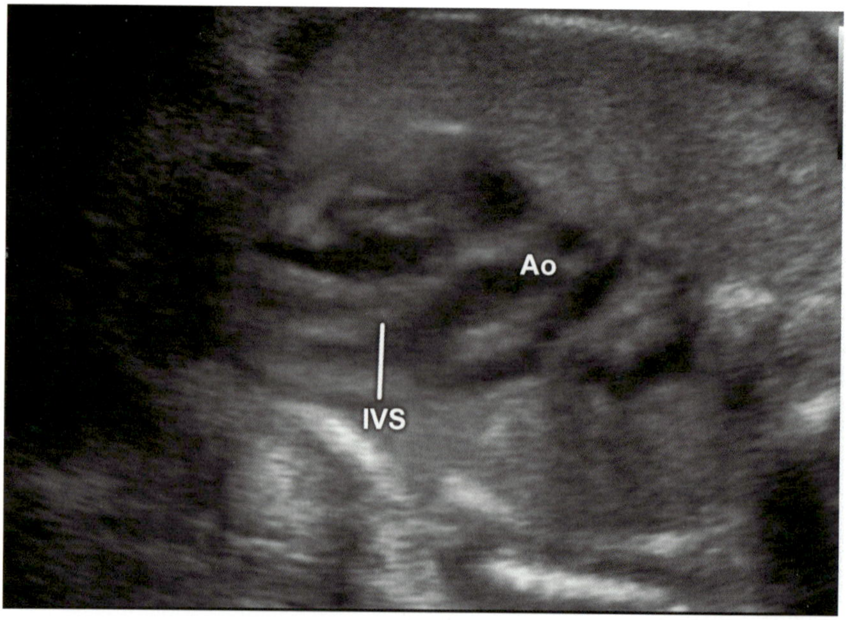

Fig. 15

5. The ascending aorta forms the transverse aortic arch after it traverses between the two atria (Fig. 16).

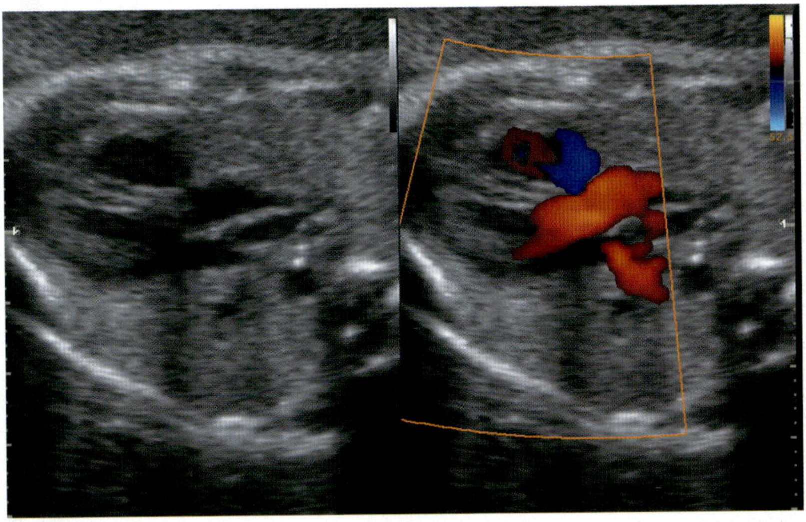

Fig. 16

6. The superior wall of the ascending aorta is continuous with the interventricular septum (Fig. 17).

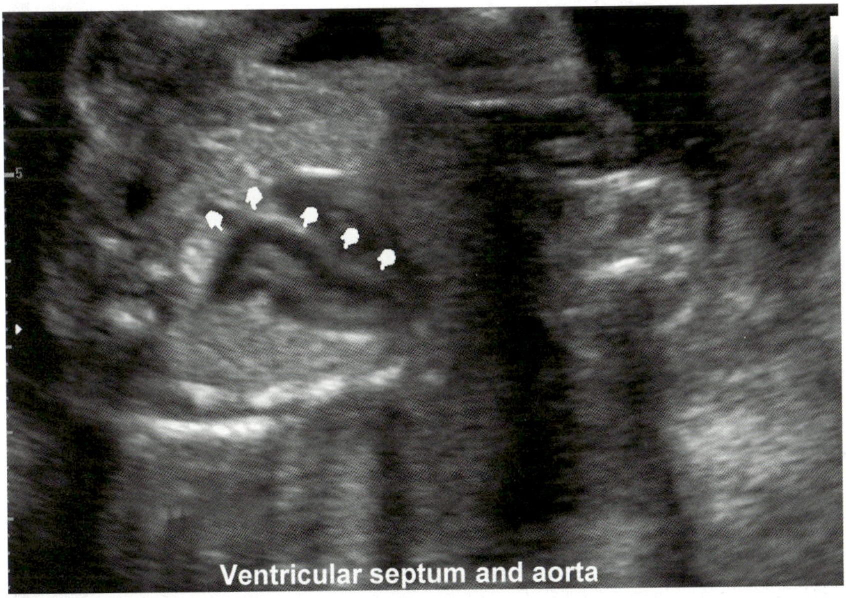

Fig. 17

7. The posterior wall of the aorta is continuous with the left atrioventricular valve (Fig. 18).

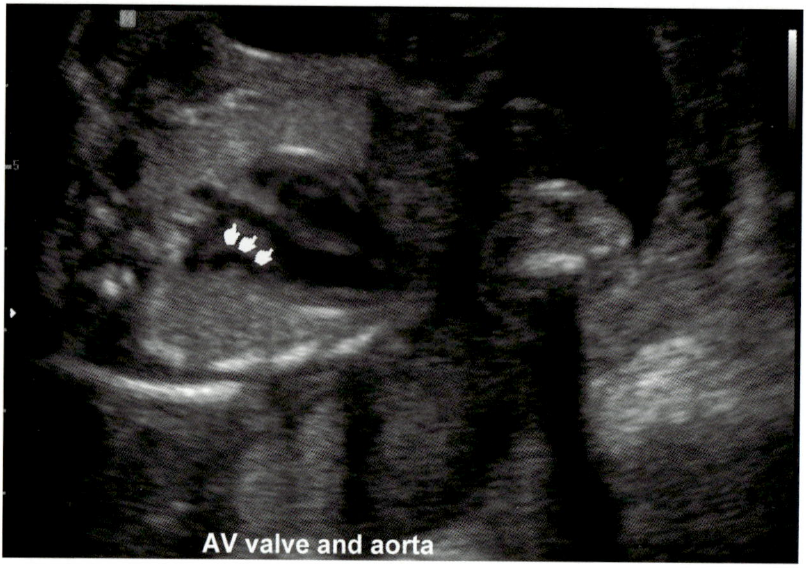

Fig. 18

8. All four chambers, the mitral valve and aorta are seen in this view. The tricuspid is not seen in the five-chamber view (Fig. 19).

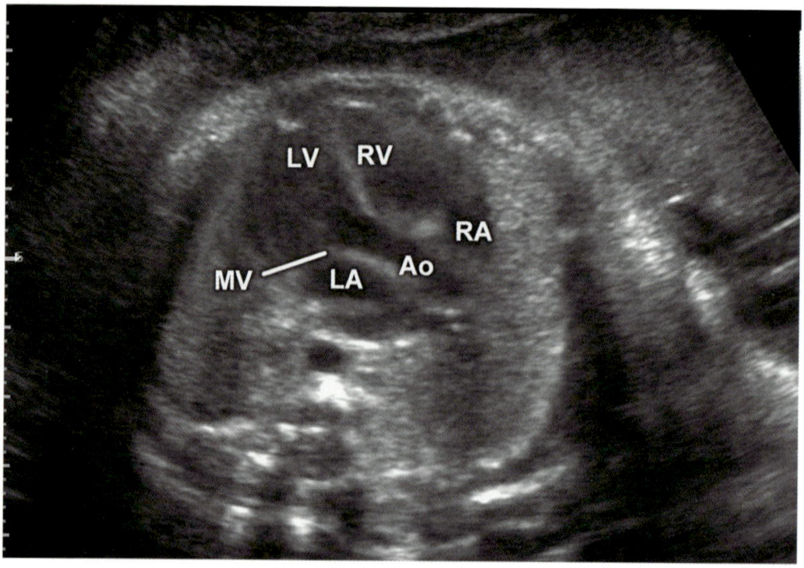

Fig. 19

Three-Vessel View

1. The three-vessel view is an extension of the transverse view superiorly in the fetal upper thorax.
2. The three-vessel view shows oblique section of the main pulmonary trunk and transverse sections of the ascending aorta and the superior vena cava.
3. The three vessels in this view are the pulmonary artery anteriorly, the superior vena cava posteriorly, and the aorta in between.
4. The pulmonary artery has the maximum diameter and the superior vena cava has the least diameter.
5. The pulmonary artery divides into the left and right pulmonary arteries where the left pulmonary artery follows the same course as the main trunk, and the right pulmonary artery traverses at a right angle posterior to the ascending aorta and the superior vena cava.

1. The three-vessel view is an extension of the transverse view superiorly in the fetal upper thorax (Figs 20A and B).

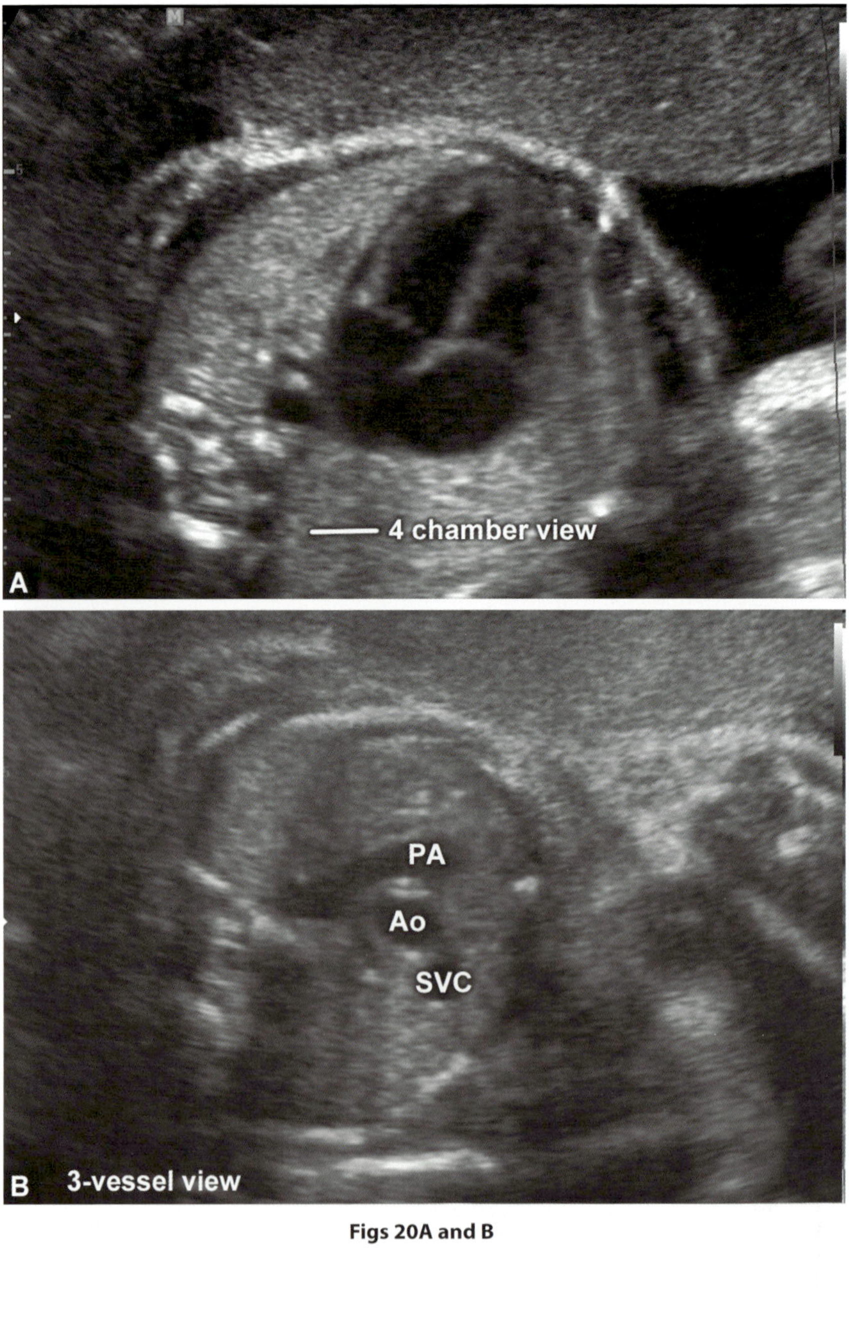

Figs 20A and B

2. The three-vessel view shows oblique section of the main pulmonary trunk and transverse sections of the ascending aorta and the superior vena cava (Fig. 21).

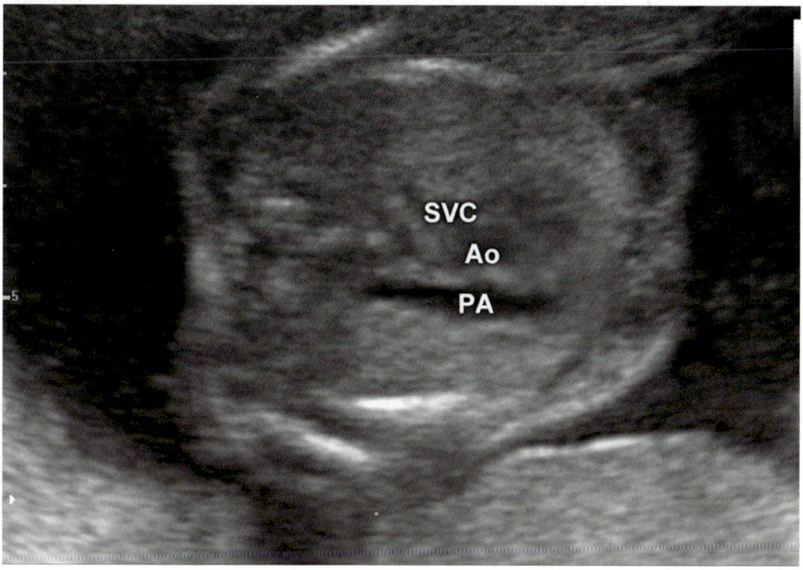

Fig. 21

3. The three vessels in this view are the pulmonary artery anteriorly, the superior vena cava posteriorly, and the aorta in between (Fig. 22).

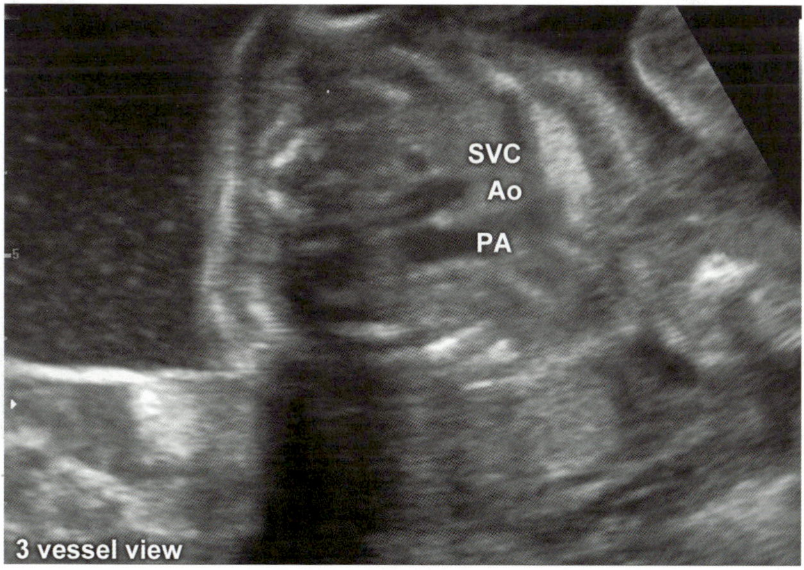

Fig. 22

4. The pulmonary artery has the maximum diameter and the superior vena cava has the least diameter (Fig. 23).

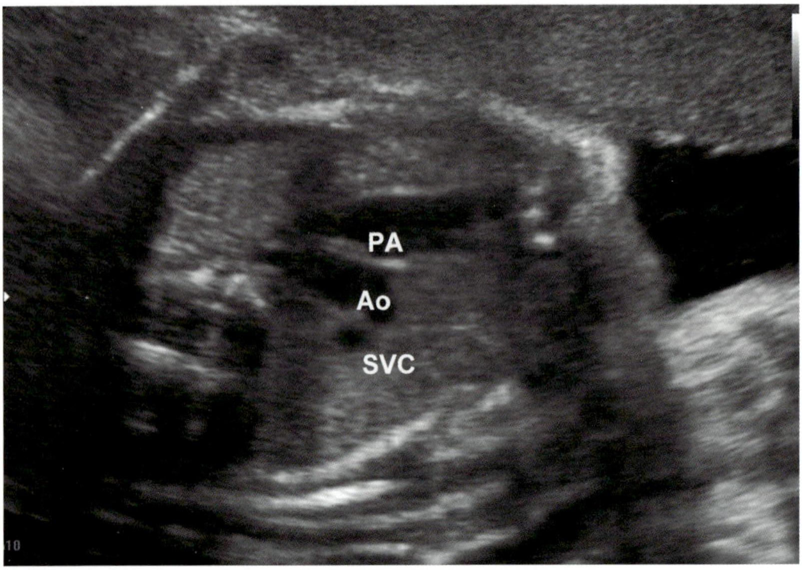

Fig. 23

5. The pulmonary artery divides into the left and right pulmonary arteries where the left pulmonary artery follows the same course as the main trunk, and the right pulmonary artery traverses at a right angle posterior to the ascending aorta and the superior vena cava (Fig. 24).

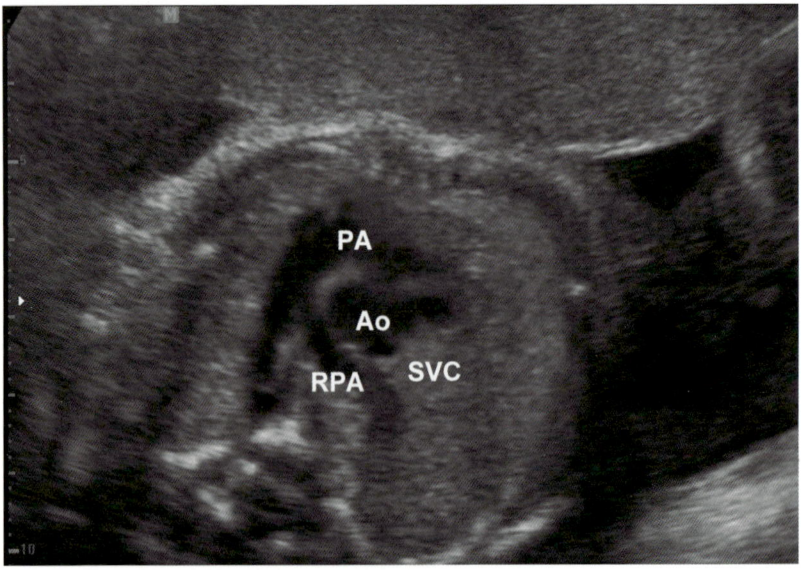

Fig. 24

Transverse Arterial Duct View

1. Tilt your transducer little cranially from your three-vessel view to get this plane.
2. You will see the main pulmonary artery with the ductal branch joining the descending aorta to the left of the spine.
3. The ascending aorta and superior vena cava will be seen on the right side in a cross-section.
4. The arrangement of these vessels with their size is the same as what you seen in the three-vessel view.

1. Tilt your transducer little cranially from your three-vessel view to get this plane (Fig. 25).

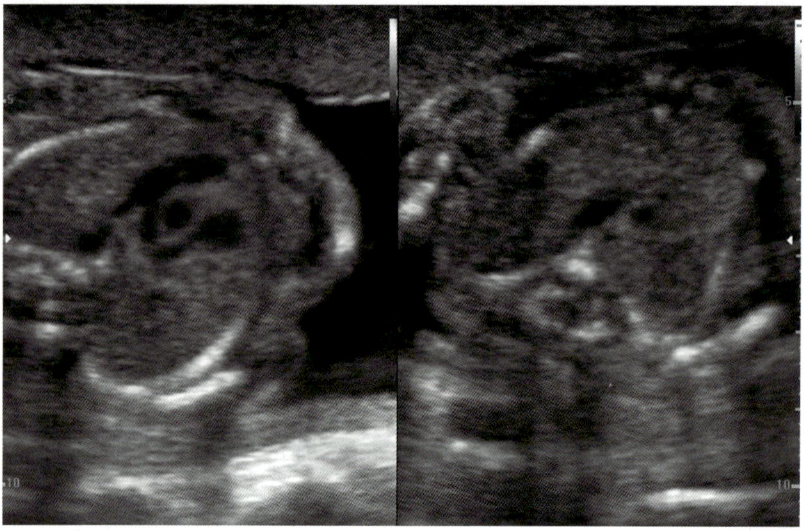

Fig. 25

2. You will see the main pulmonary artery with the ductal branch joining the descending aorta to the left of the spine (Fig. 26).

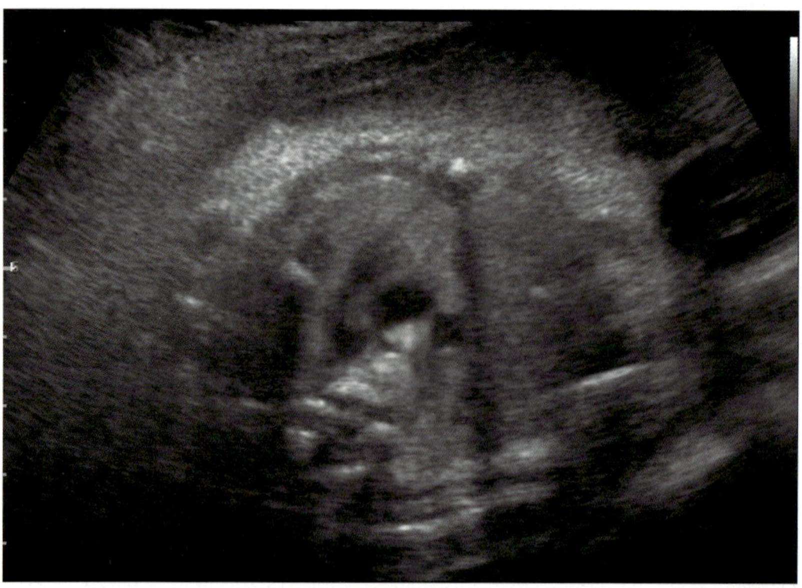

Fig. 26

3. The ascending aorta and superior vena cava will be seen on the right side in a cross section (Fig. 27).

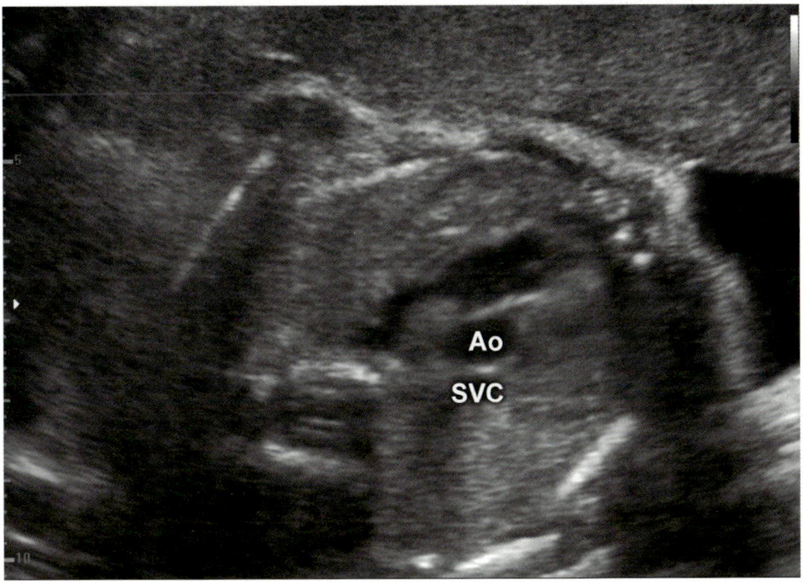

Fig. 27

4. The arrangement of these vessels with their size is the same as what you seen in the three-vessel view (Fig. 28).

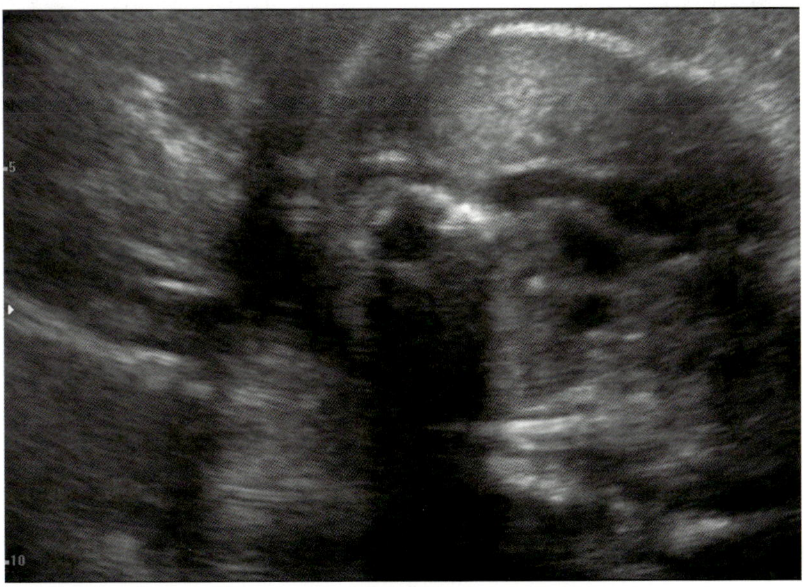

Fig. 28

Aortic Arch Transverse View

1. From the transverse arterial duct view slide your transducer cranially to get this view. You see the transverse aortic arch, which is the most superior vessel in the thorax.
2. You see two vessels in this view: the transverse aortic arch and the superior vena cava.

1. From the transverse arterial duct view slide your transducer cranially to get this view. You see the transverse aortic arch, which is the most superior vessel in the thorax (Fig. 29).

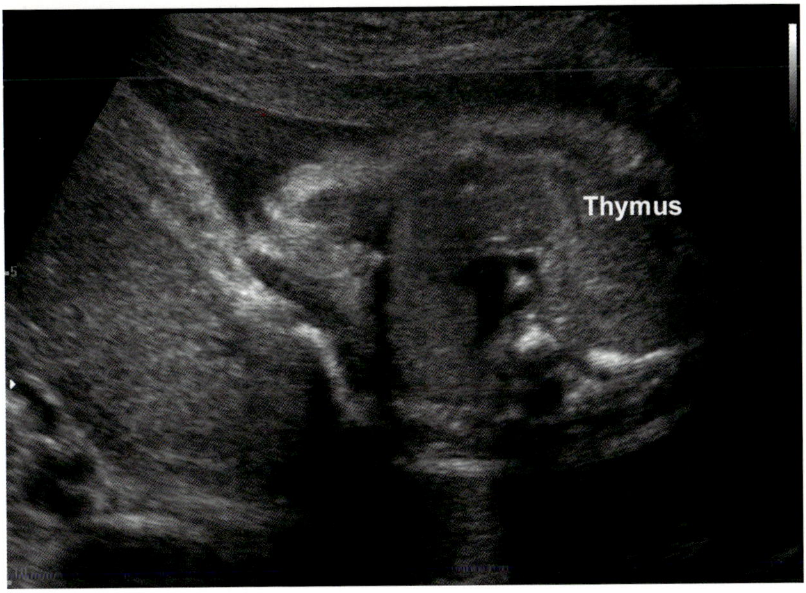

Fig. 29

2. You see two vessels in this view: the transverse aortic arch and the superior vena cava (Fig. 30).

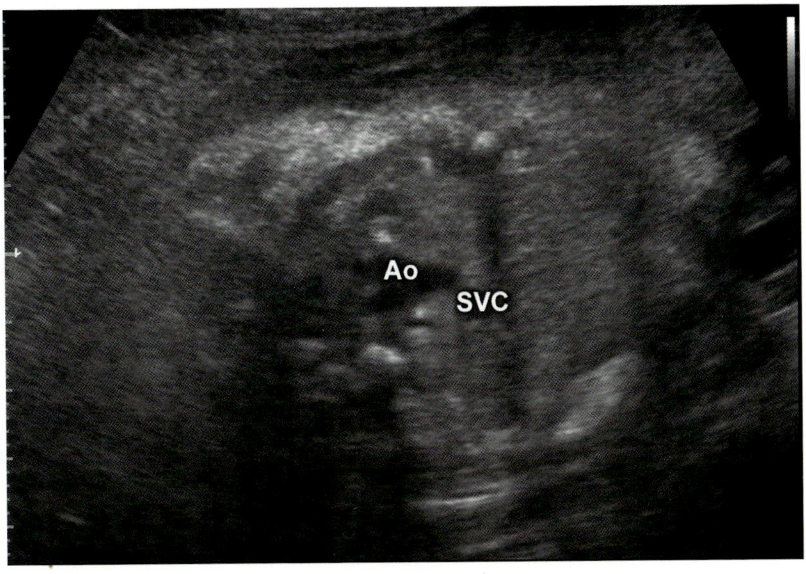

Fig. 30

Three-Vessel Trachea View

1. This view is more cranial to the three-vessel view. It shows the aortic arch and ductal arch merging together into the descending aorta with an acute angle between them.
2. The aortic and ductal arches are seen to the left of the spine and trachea. This is an important anatomic marker as you do not see any vessel to the right of the trachea.

1. This view is more cranial to the three-vessel view. It shows the aortic arch and ductal arch merging together into the descending aorta with an acute angle between them (Fig. 31).

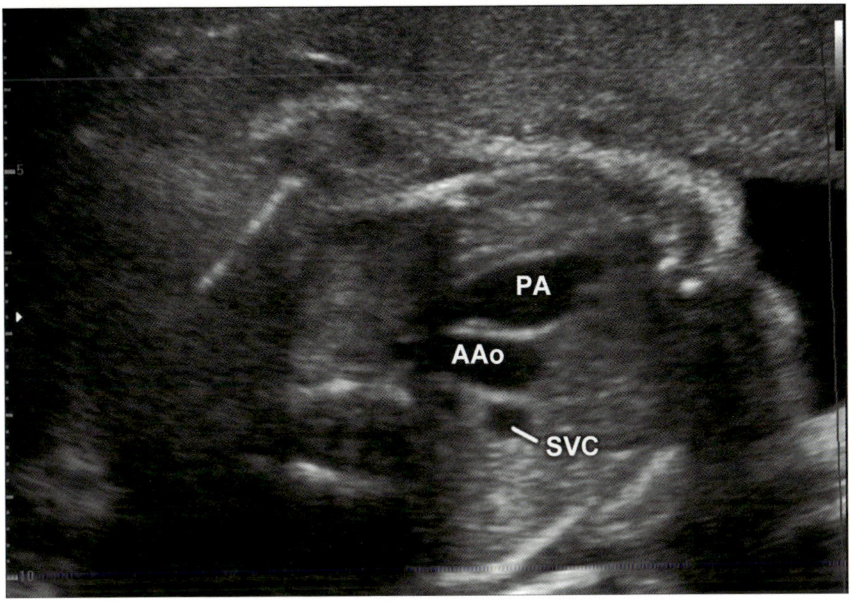

Fig. 31

2. The aortic and ductal arches are seen to the left of the spine and trachea. This is an important anatomic marker as you do not see any vessel to the right of the trachea (Fig. 32).

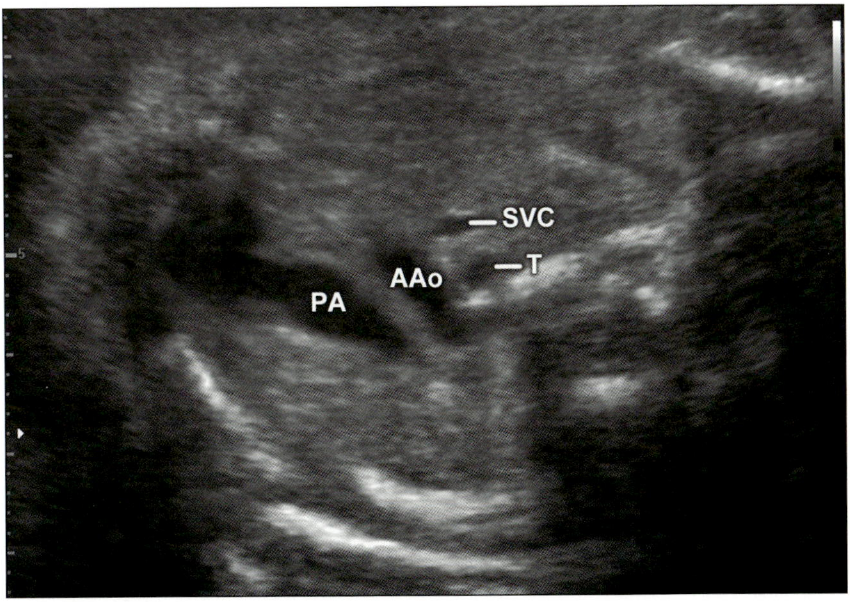

Fig. 32

SAGITTAL VIEW

1. Ascertain the fetal situs.
2. View the fetal thorax and take a sagittal view of the fetal spine in the thoracic region.
3. Rock your transducer from the right parasagittal to the left parasagittal plane and view the caval veins, aortic arch and ductal arch from right to left.
4. Be patient for good views with the spine posterior rather than anterior or on the lateral aspect.
5. The bicaval view is seen in the right parasagittal plane showing the inferior and superior venae cavae entering the posterior aspect of the right atrium.
6. From the bicaval view slide your transducer to the left side and you see the aorta arising from the central portion of the fetal heart making an arch called the aortic arch. This looks like a candy or a walking cane. From the superior aspect of the aortic arch three vessels are seen arising from it.
7. On sliding your transducer further to the left you see the ductal arch arising from the anterior most chamber with a wide curvature. The ductal arch does not give any branches and connects with the descending aorta. The ductal arch represents an ice hockey stick.

1. Ascertain the fetal situs (Fig. 33).

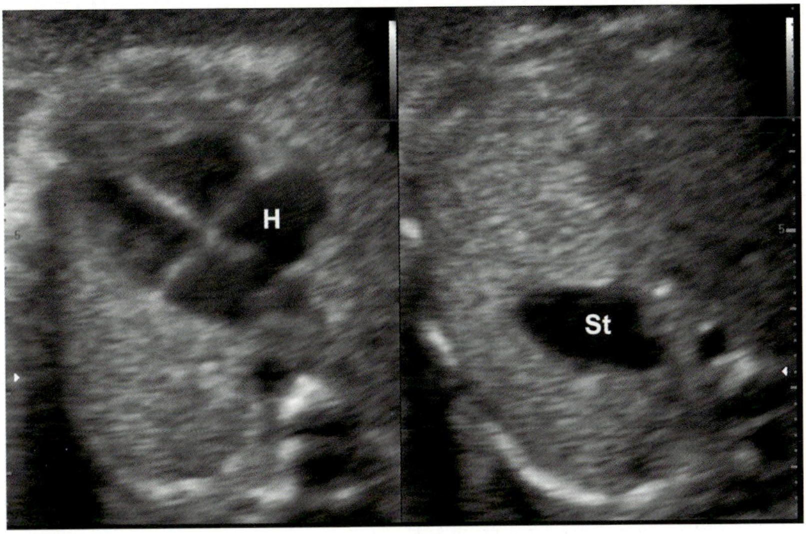

Fig. 33

2. View the fetal thorax and take a sagittal view of the fetal spine in the thoracic region (Fig. 34).

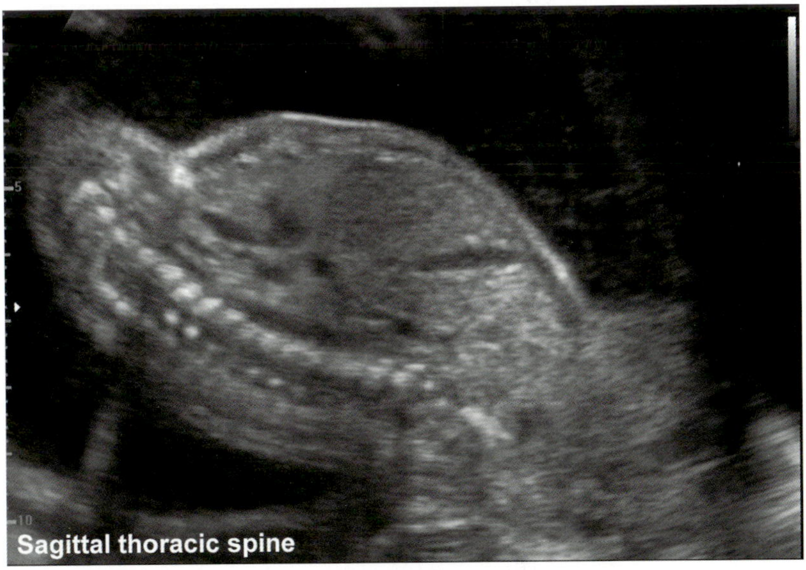

Fig. 34

3. Rock your transducer from the right parasagittal to the left parasagittal plane and view the caval veins, aortic arch and ductal arch from right to left (Fig. 35).

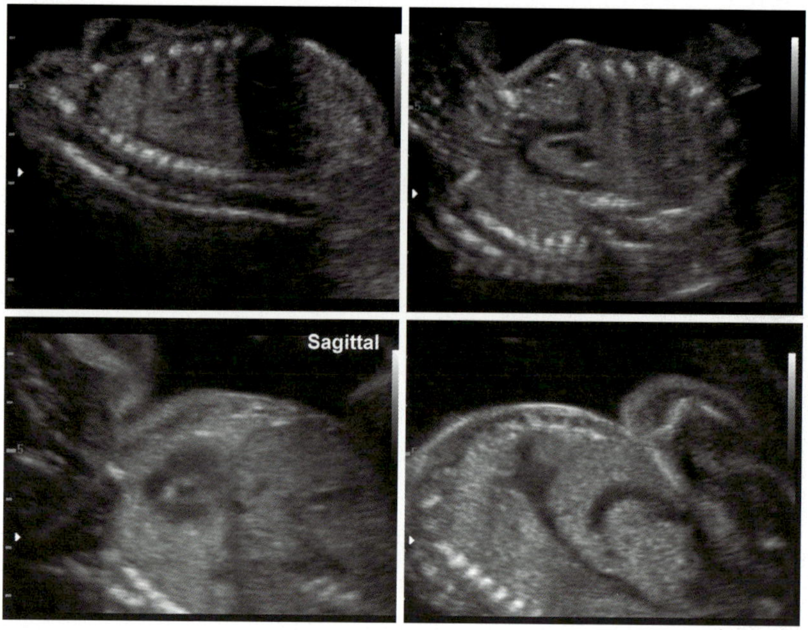

Fig. 35

4. Be patient for good views with the spine posterior rather than anterior or on the lateral aspect (Fig. 36).

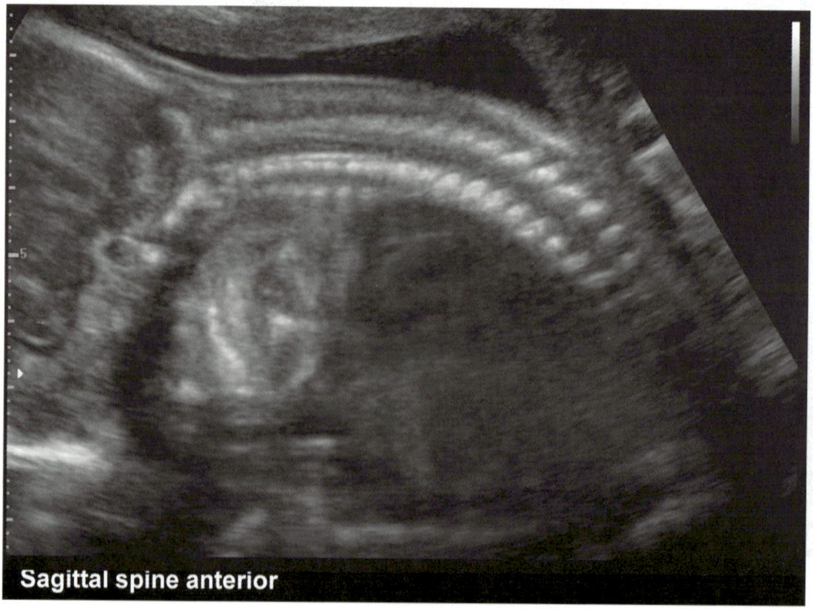

Fig. 36

5. The bicaval view is seen in the right parasagittal plane showing the inferior and superior venae cavae entering the posterior aspect of the right atrium (Figs 37A and B).

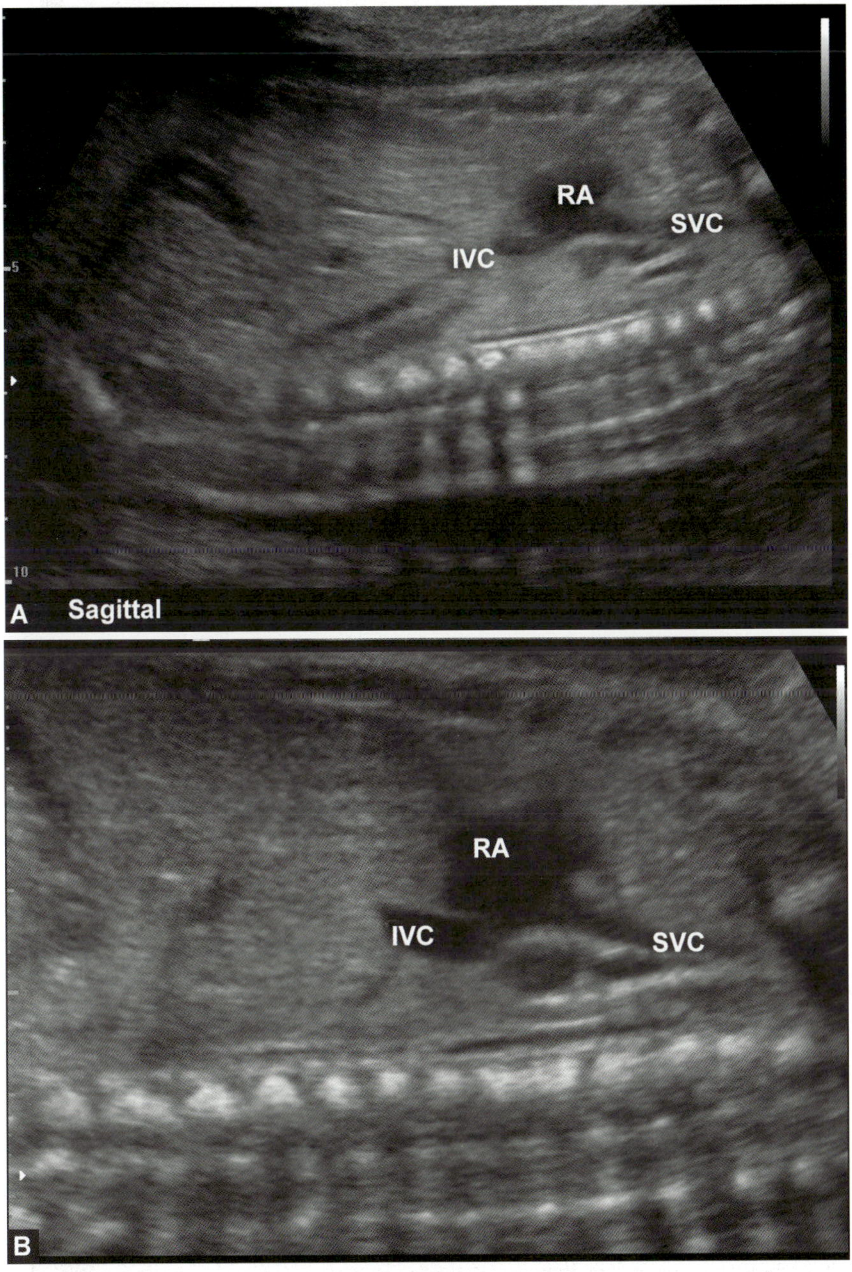

Figs 37A and B

6. From the bicaval view slide your transducer to the left side and you see the aorta arising from the central portion of the fetal heart making an arch called the aortic arch. This looks like a candy or a walking cane. From the superior aspect of the aortic arch three vessels are seen arising from it (Figs 38A and B).

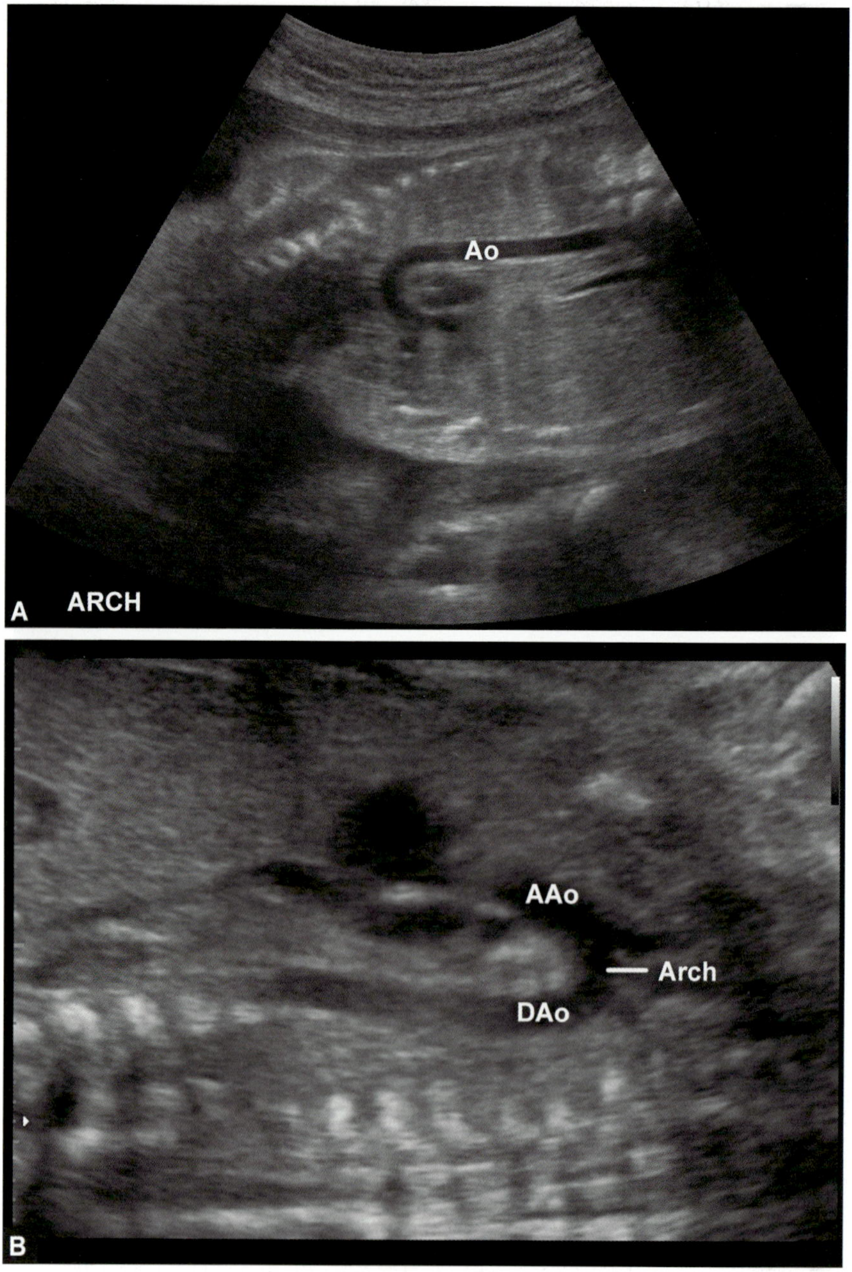

Figs 38A and B

7. On sliding your transducer further to the left you see the ductal arch arising from the anterior most chamber with a wide curvature. The ductal arch does not give any branches and connects with the descending aorta. The ductal arch represents an ice hockey stick (Figs 39A and B).

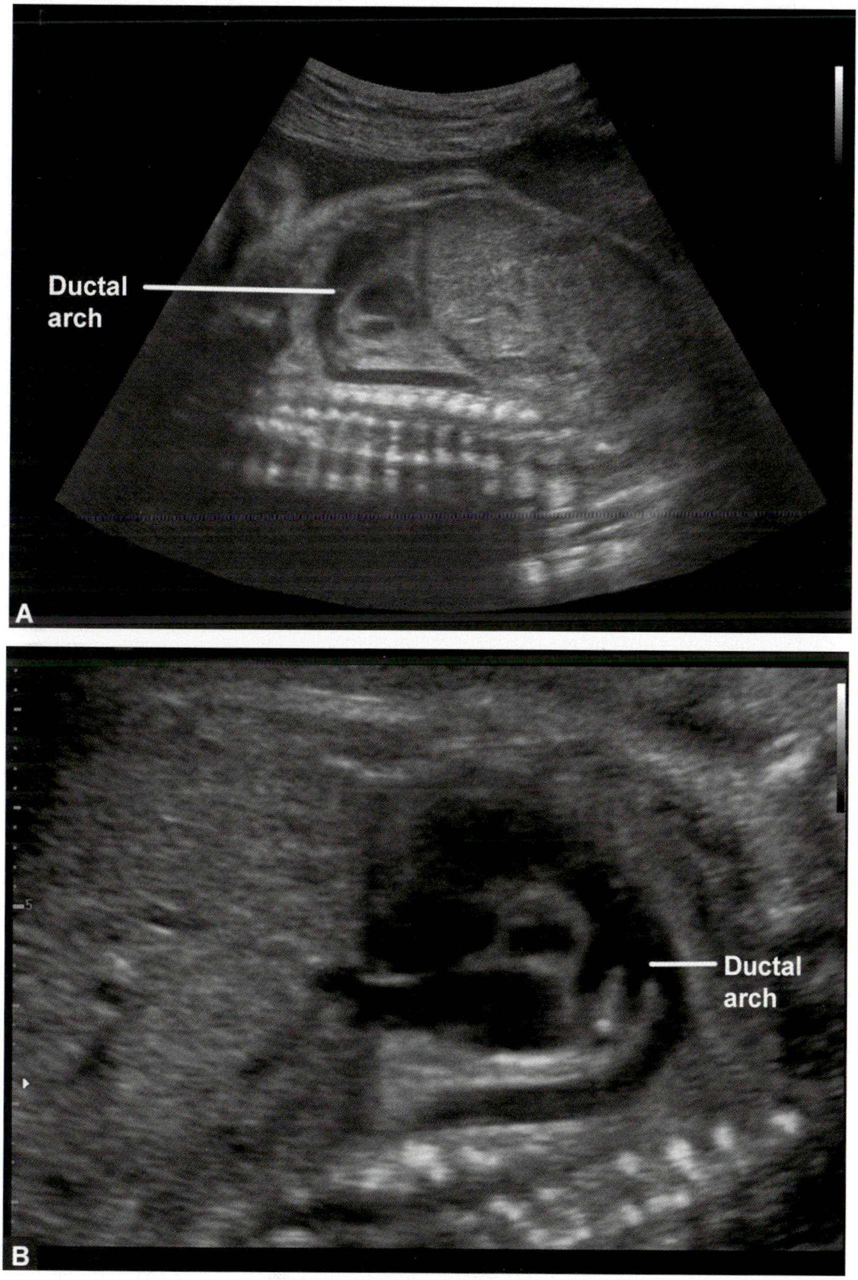

Figs 39A and B

Bicaval View

1. The bicaval view is obtained in a right parasagittal plane.
2. This plane shows the inferior and superior vena cava entering the posterior aspect of the right atrium.

1. The bicaval view is obtained in a right parasagittal plane (Fig. 40).

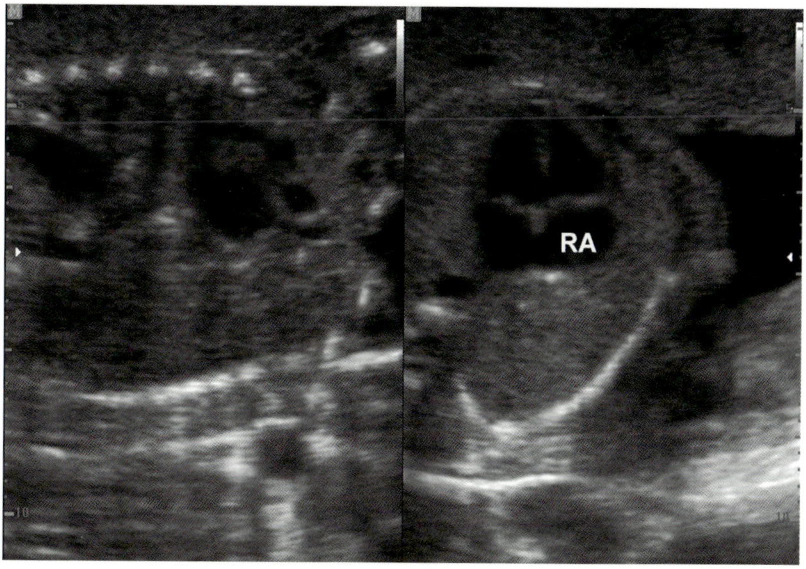

Fig. 40

2. This plane shows the inferior and superior vena cava entering the posterior aspect of the right atrium (Fig. 41).

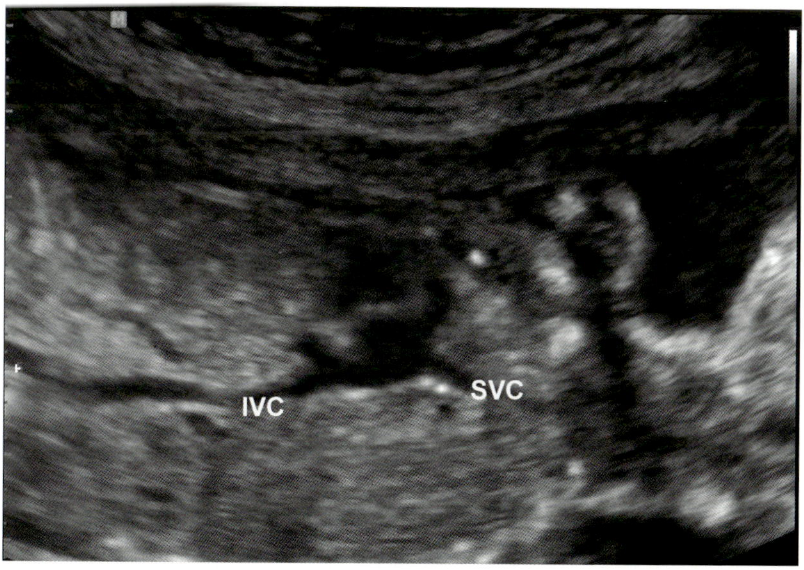

Fig. 41

Aortic Arch View

1. The ascending aorta arises from the left ventricle in the central portion of the heart.
2. The ascending aorta angles anteriorly, pointing towards the fetal right shoulder and parallel to the long-axis of the left ventricle as it comes out of the heart.
3. The ascending aorta is continuous anteriorly with the interventricular septum. The continuity between the anterior wall of the ascending aorta and the interventricular septum is helpful in excluding outlet VSD.
4. The ascending aorta is continuous posteriorly with the anterior leaflet of the mitral valve.
5. The ascending aorta extends between the right and left atrium and runs inferior to the pulmonary artery.
6. There are three arterial branches of the aortic arch: the brachiocephalic (innominate), the left common carotid, and the left subclavian artery. The aortic arch provides the majority of blood supply to the head, neck, and upper extremities. The aortic arch branching provide an important clue to distinguish the aortic arch from the ductal arch, which gives no branches as it connects with the descending aorta.
7. During left ventricular diastole, blood does not flow back into the ventricle by the aortic semilunar valve.

1. The ascending aorta arises from the left ventricle in the central portion of the heart (Figs 42A and B).

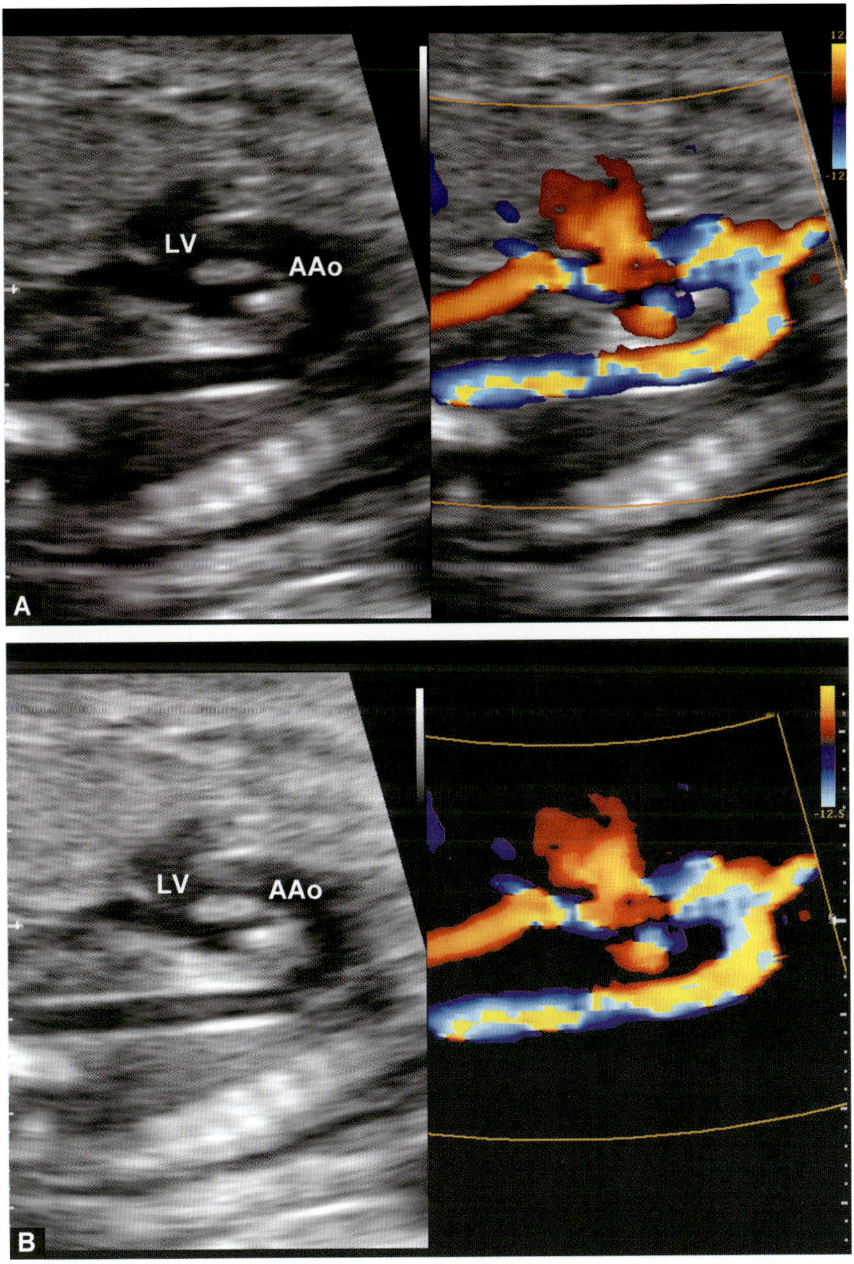

Figs 42A and B

2. The ascending aorta angles anteriorly, pointing towards the fetal right shoulder and parallel to the long-axis of the left ventricle as it comes out of the heart (Fig. 43).

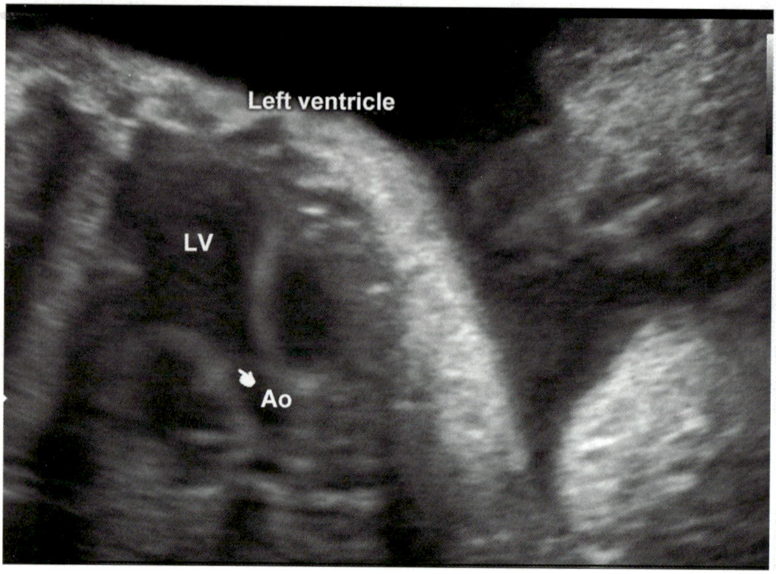

Fig. 43

3. The ascending aorta is continuous anteriorly with the interventricular septum. The continuity between the anterior wall of the ascending aorta and the interventricular septum is helpful in excluding outlet VSD (Fig. 44).

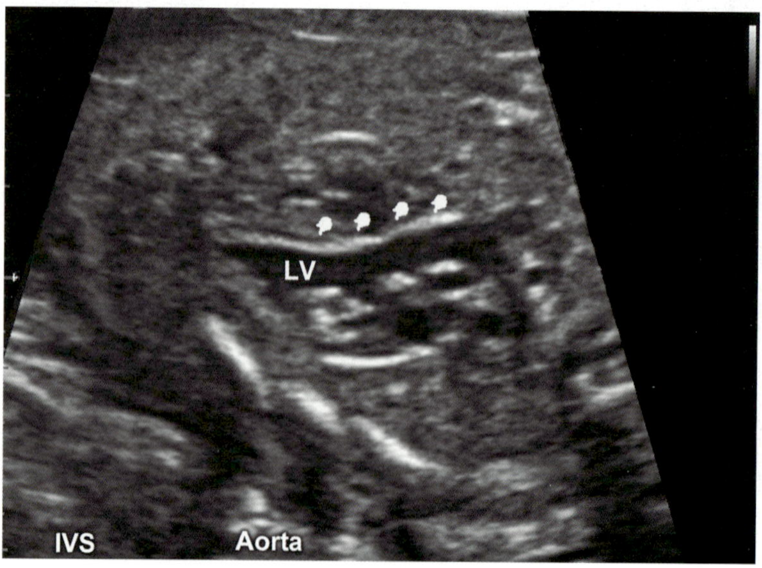

Fig. 44

4. The ascending aorta is continuous posteriorly with the anterior leaflet of the mitral valve (Fig. 45).

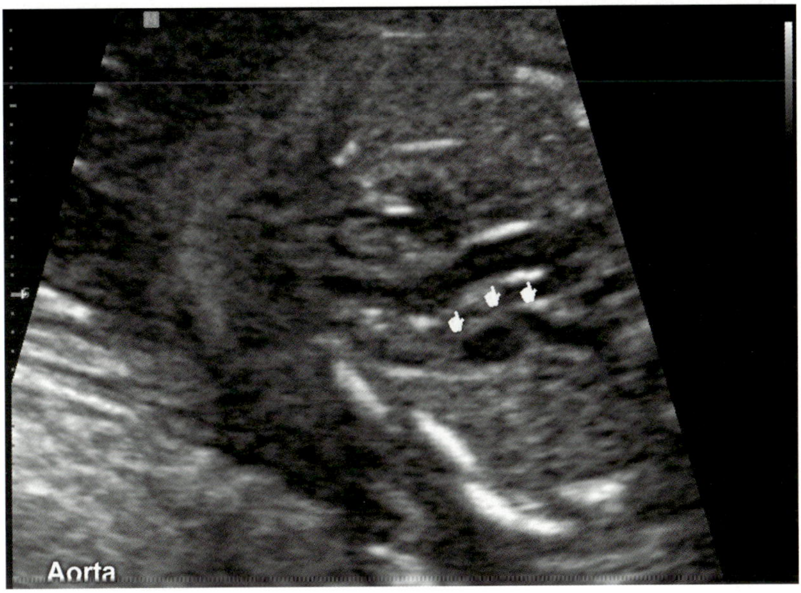

Fig. 45

5. The ascending aorta extends between the right and left atrium and runs inferior to the pulmonary artery (Figs 46A and B).

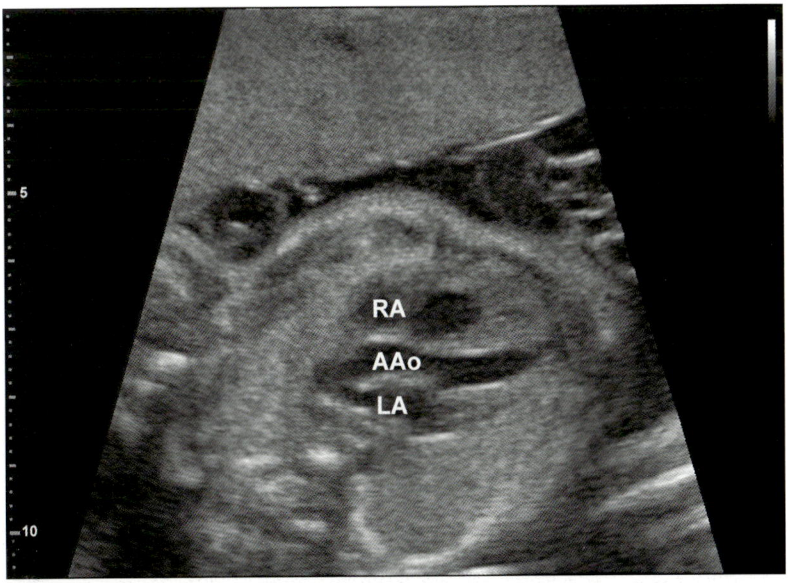

Fig. 46A

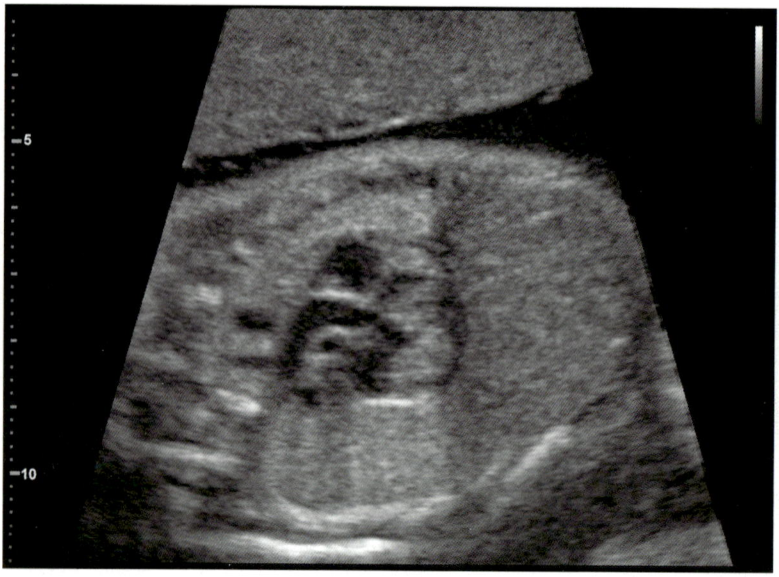

Fig. 46B

6. There are three arterial branches of the aortic arch: the brachiocephalic (innominate), the left common carotid, and the left subclavian artery. The aortic arch provides the majority of blood supply to the head, neck, and upper extremities. The aortic arch branching provide an important clue to distinguish the aortic arch from the ductal arch, which gives no branches as it connects with the descending aorta (Figs 47A and B).

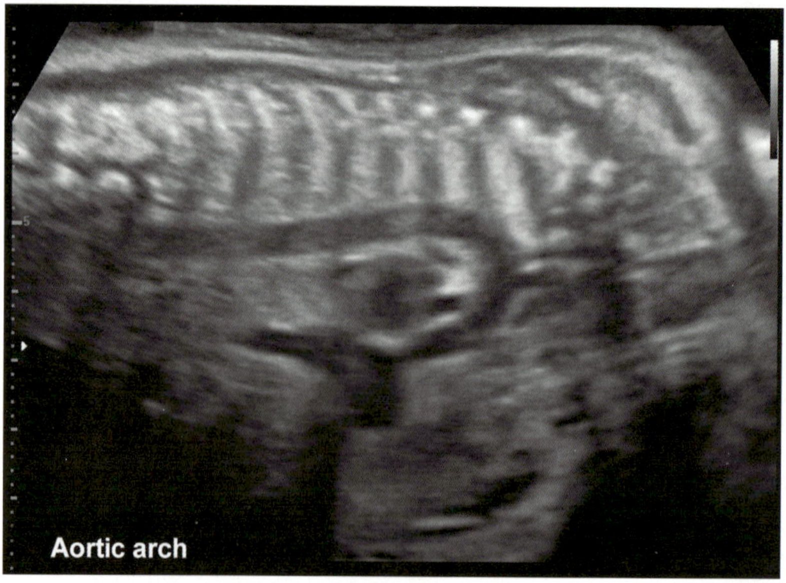

Fig. 47A

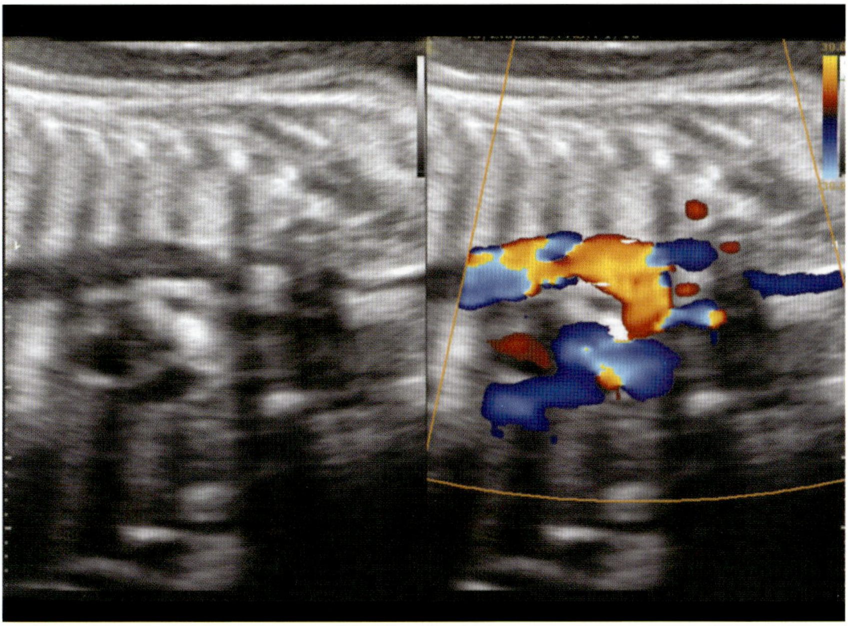

Fig. 47B

7. During left ventricular diastole, blood does not flow back into the ventricle by the aortic semilunar valve (Fig. 48).

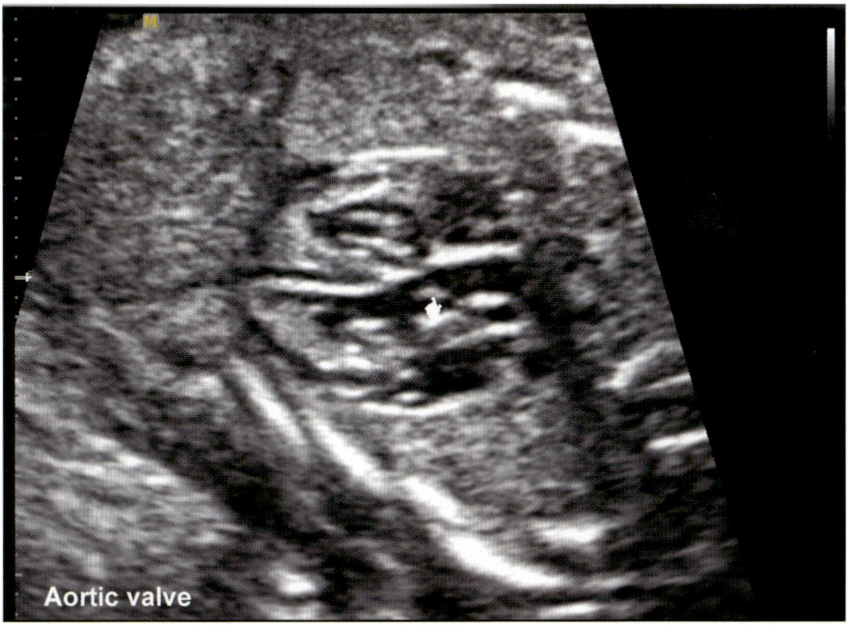

Fig. 48

Ductal Arch View

1. The pulmonary artery (main pulmonary artery, pulmonary trunk) originates from the right ventricle in the anterior aspect of the fetal heart.
2. The pulmonary artery crosses over the aorta and points toward the fetal left shoulder as it emerges from the right ventricle.
3. The pulmonary artery, shortly after crossing over the aorta, dips posteriorly into the chest dividing into the right and left pulmonary arteries and the ductus arteriosus.
4. The ductus arteriosus, is patent in the fetus, then connects with the descending aorta.
5. The division of the pulmonary artery into the right and left pulmonary arteries differentiates it from the ascending aorta.
6. The left pulmonary artery continues posteriorly and inferiorly.
7. The right pulmonary artery originates at a right angle from the pulmonary artery and crosses posterior to the aortic arch, superior to the roof of the left atrium and behind the superior vena cava, before dipping into the right lung hilum.
8. During right ventricular diastole, blood does not flow back into the ventricle by the pulmonary semilunar valve.

1. The pulmonary artery (main pulmonary artery, pulmonary trunk) originates from the right ventricle in the anterior aspect of the fetal heart (Figs 49A and B).

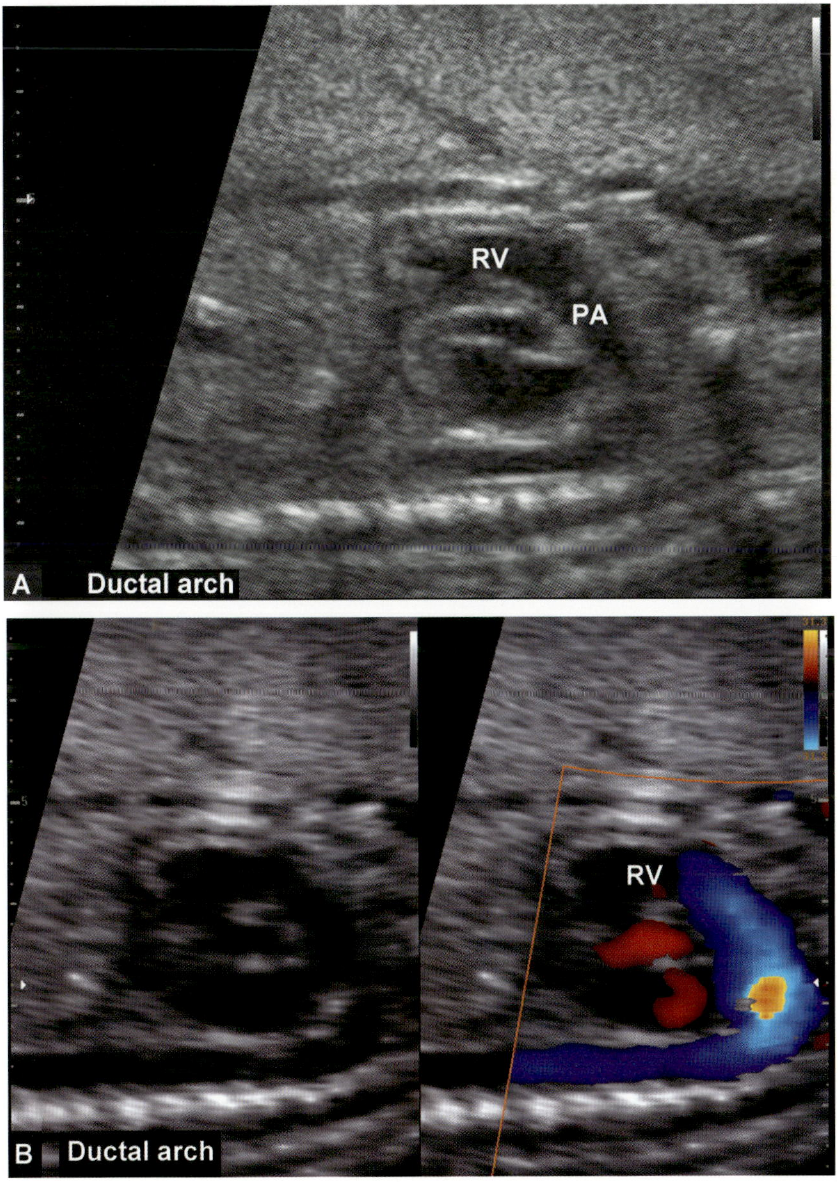

Figs 49A and B

2. The pulmonary artery crosses over the aorta and points toward the fetal left shoulder as it emerges from the right ventricle (Fig. 50).

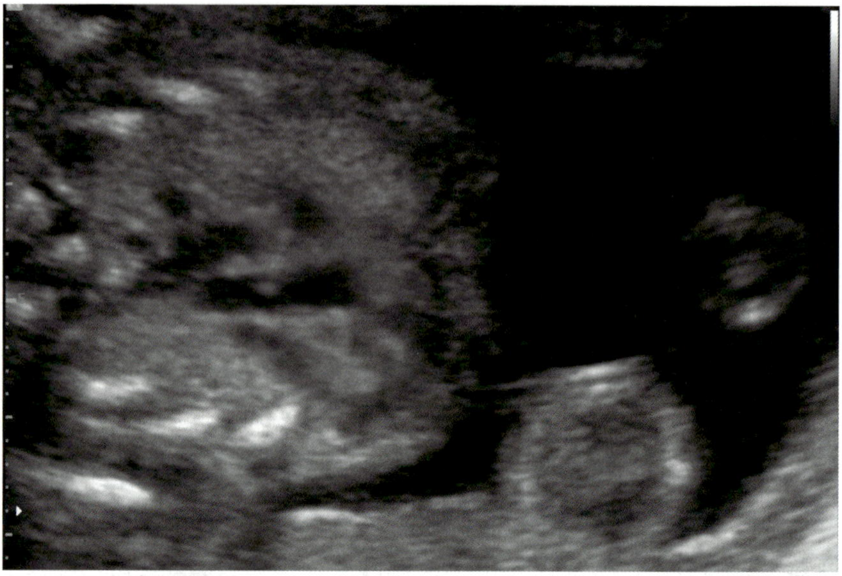

Fig. 50

3. The pulmonary artery, shortly after crossing over the aorta, dips posteriorly into the chest dividing into the right and left pulmonary arteries and the ductus arteriosus (Fig. 51).

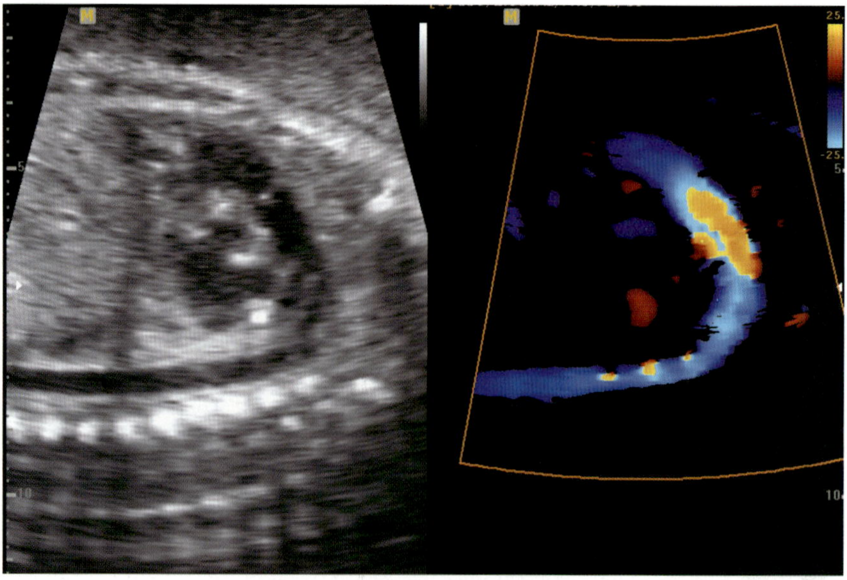

Fig. 51

4. The ductus arteriosus, is patent in the fetus, then connects with the descending aorta (Fig. 52).

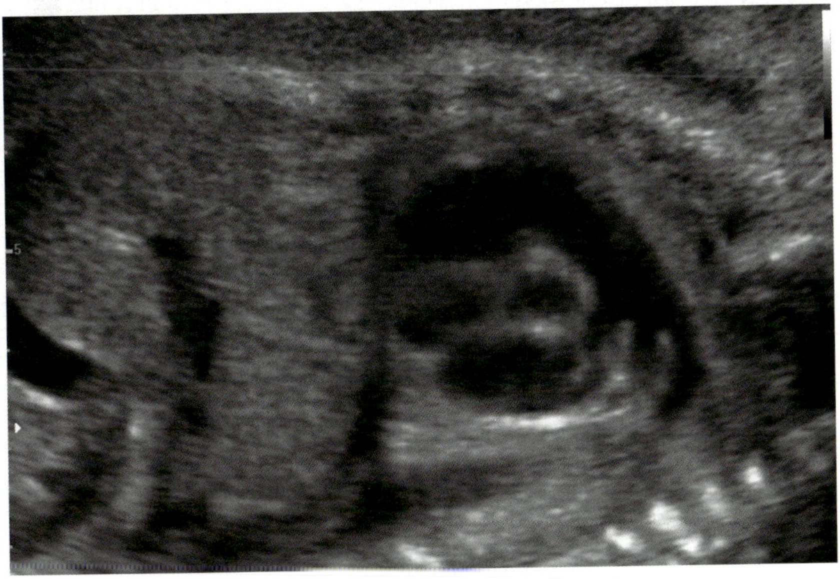

Fig. 52

5. The division of the pulmonary artery into the right and left pulmonary arteries differentiates it from the ascending aorta (Fig. 53).

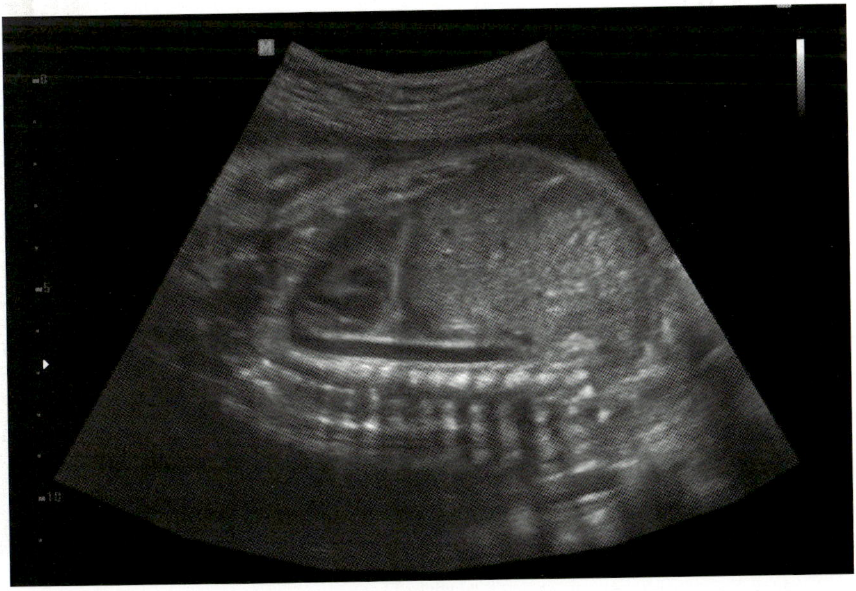

Fig. 53

6. The left pulmonary artery continues posteriorly and inferiorly (Fig. 54).

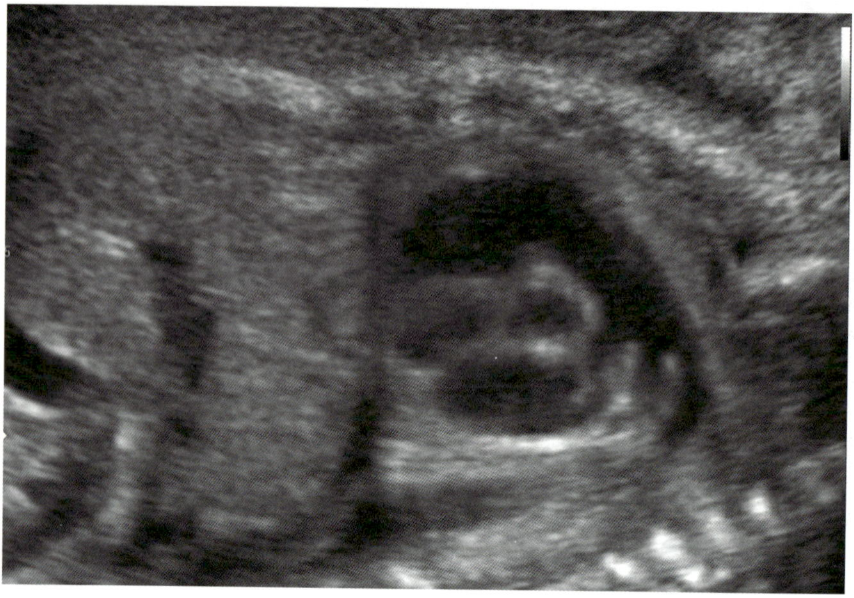

Fig. 54

7. The right pulmonary artery originates at a right angle from the pulmonary artery and crosses posterior to the aortic arch, superior to the roof of the left atrium and behind the superior vena cava, before dipping into the right lung hilum (Figs 55A and B).

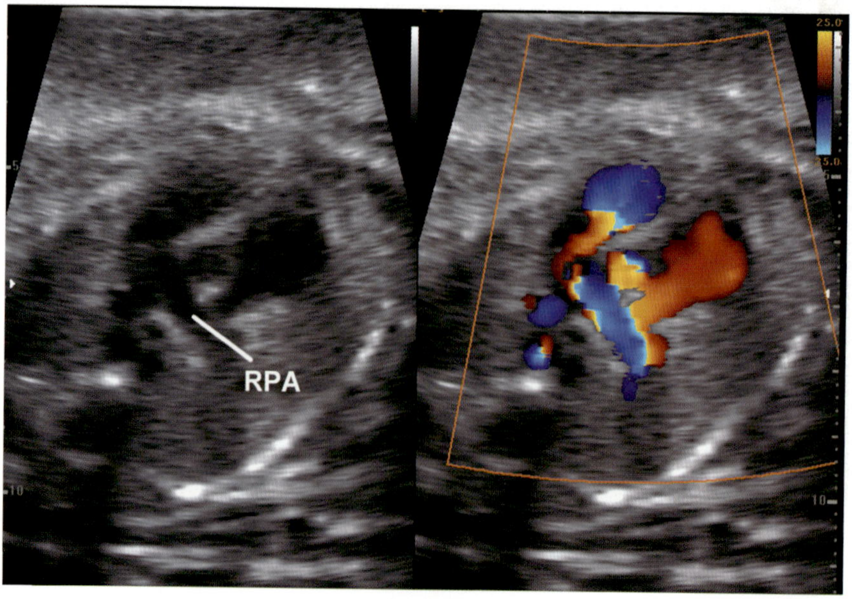

Fig. 55A

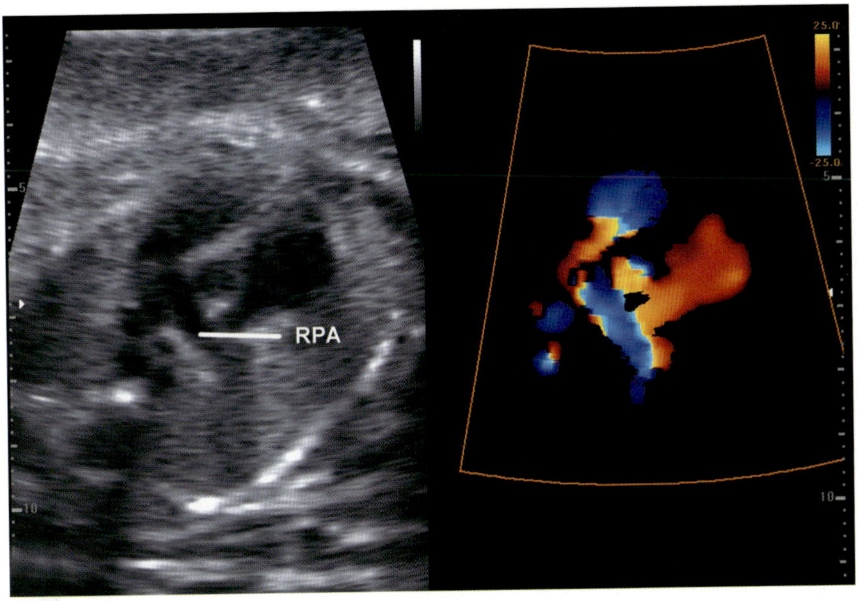

Fig. 55B

8. During right ventricular diastole, blood does not flow back into the ventricle by the pulmonary semilunar valve (Fig. 56).

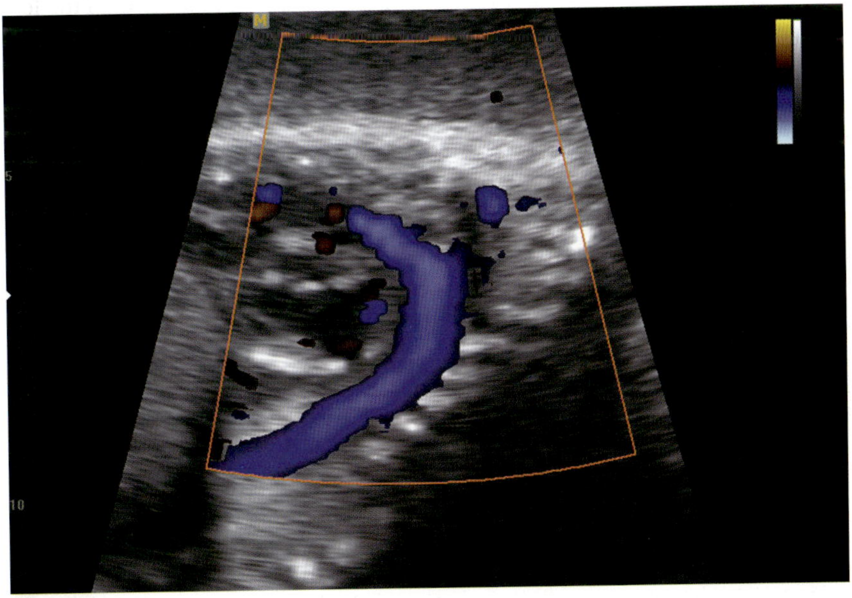

Fig. 56

OBLIQUE

Right Ventricular Outflow View

1. In this view, the right ventricular inflow and outflow tracts can be seen in the same plane.
2. The main pulmonary artery is seen and it crosses over the aorta and divides into the right pulmonary artery and ductus arteriosus.
3. The right pulmonary artery posterior to the aorta and to the right side. The aorta is seen in a cross section at the level of the aortic valve.

1. In this view, the right ventricular inflow and outflow tracts can be seen in the same plane (Fig. 57).

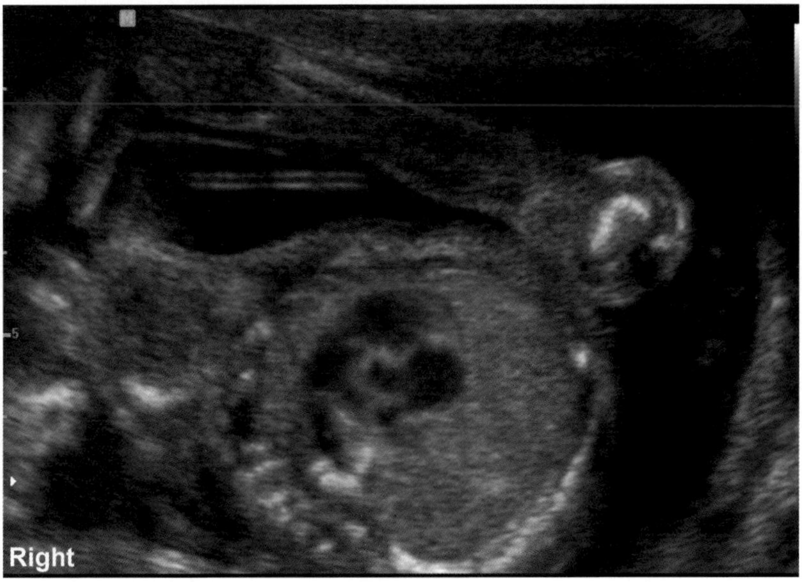

Fig. 57

2. The main pulmonary artery is seen and it crosses over the aorta and divides into the right pulmonary artery and ductus arteriosus (Fig. 58).

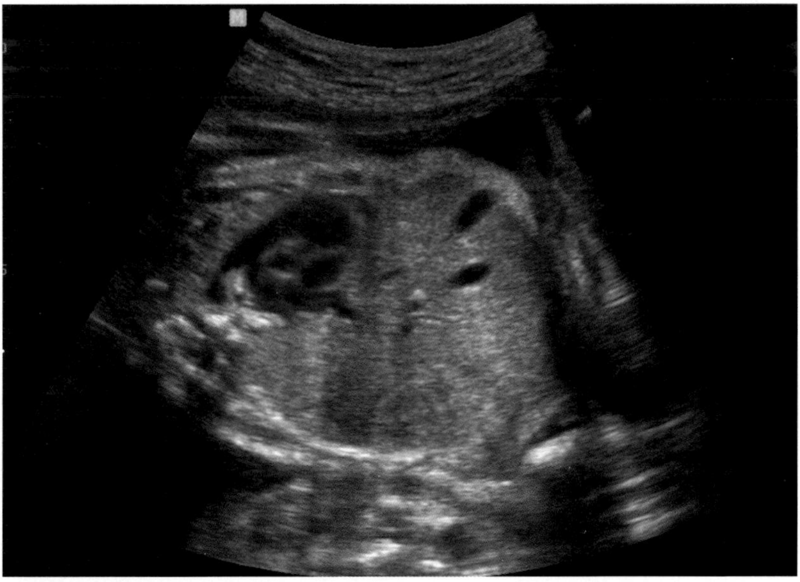

Fig. 58

3. The right pulmonary artery posterior to the aorta and to the right side. The aorta is seen in a cross section at the level of the aortic valve (Fig. 59).

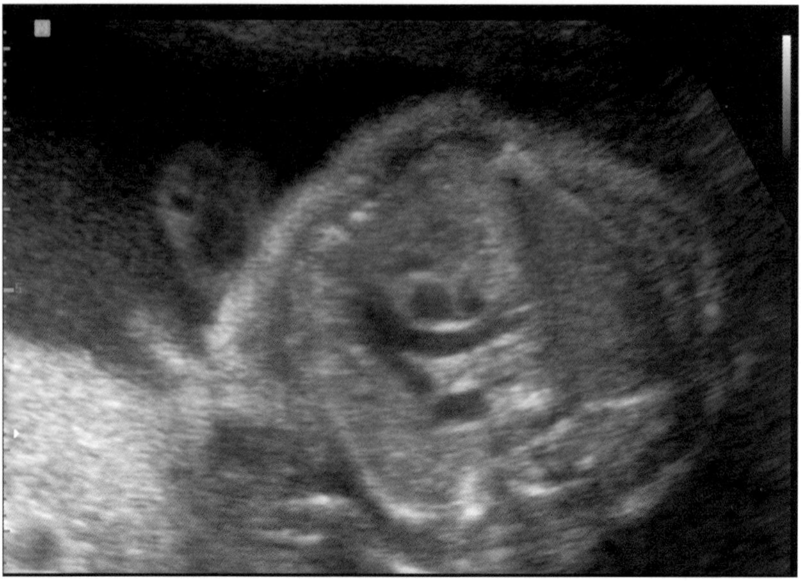

Fig. 59

Left Ventricular Long-Axis View

1. The anterior wall continuity of the aorta with the ventricular septum and the continuity of the posterior wall of the aorta with the anterior leaflet of the mitral valve are delineated.
2. The perimembranous and muscular parts of the ventricular septum are seen.
3. The inflow and outflow tracts of the left ventricle have a much narrower angle than those of the right ventricle which has a more perpendicular orientation.

1. The anterior wall continuity of the aorta with the ventricular septum and the continuity of the posterior wall of the aorta with the anterior leaflet of the mitral valve are delineated (Figs 60A and B).

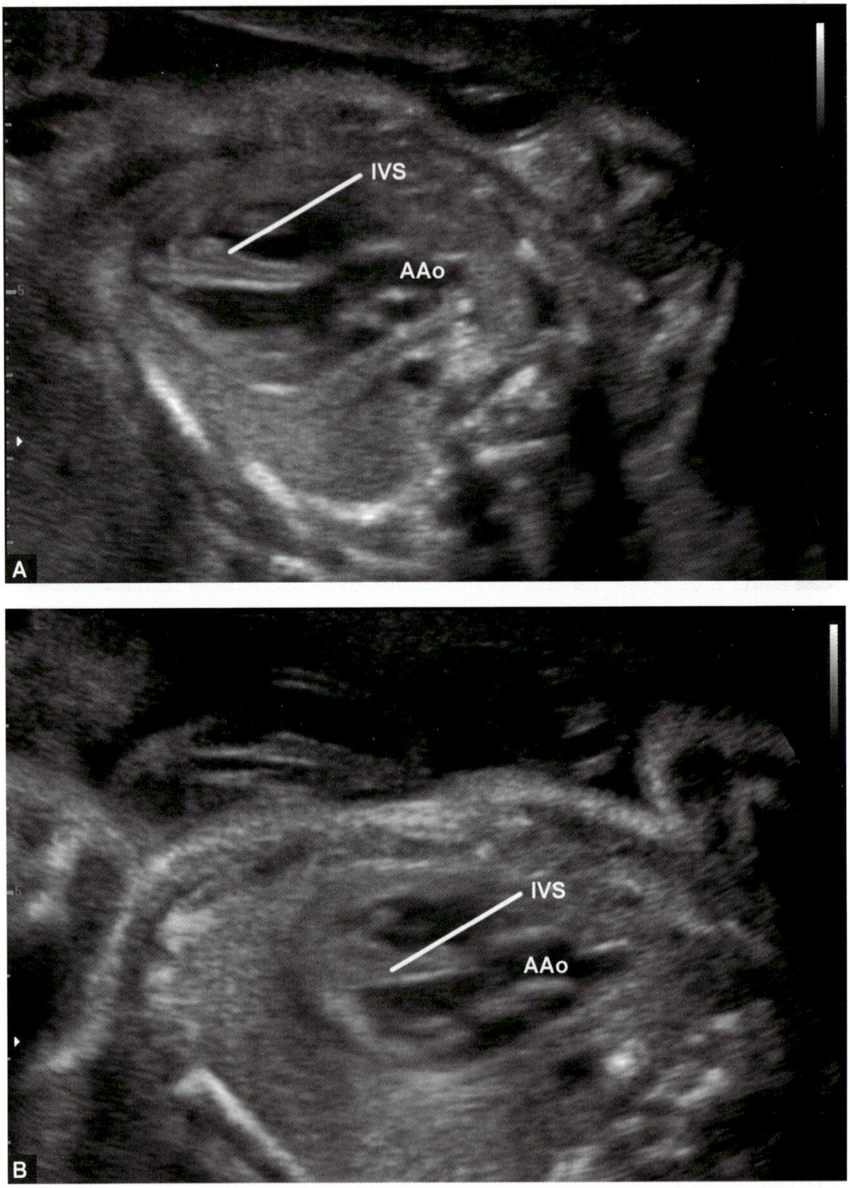

Figs 60A and B

2. The perimembranous and muscular parts of the ventricular septum are seen (Fig. 61).

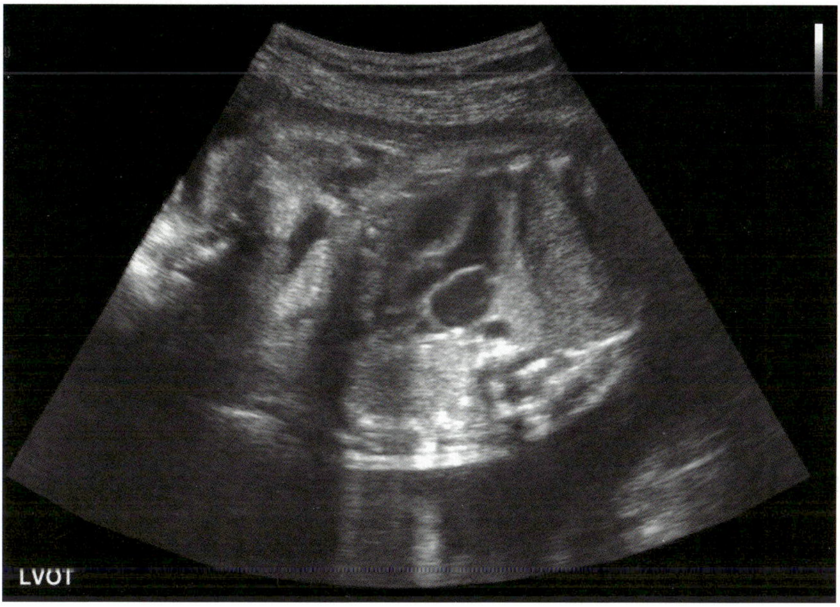

Fig. 61

3. The inflow and outflow tracts of the left ventricle have a much narrower angle than those of the right ventricle which has a more perpendicular orientation (Fig. 62).

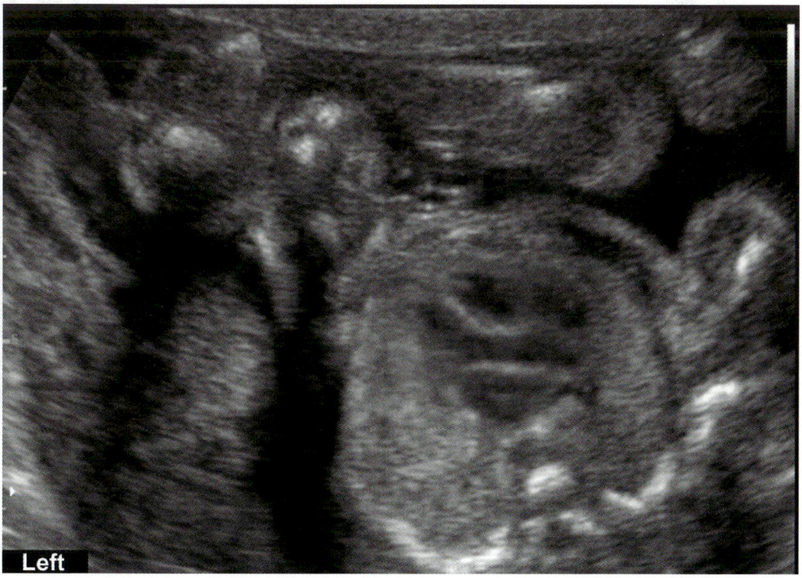

Fig. 62

Ventricular Short-Axis View

1. From the four-chamber view, plane rotates the transducer 90 degree to get the short-axis views of the heart.
2. These views provide a detailed anatomic evaluation of the relationship of cardiac chambers and are also useful in the evaluation of ventricular size, ventricular wall, and septal thickness.
3. In the apical short-axis view, the left ventricle is circular in shape and posterior to the right ventricle.

1. From the four-chamber view, plane rotates the transducer 90 degree to get the short-axis views of the heart (Fig. 63).

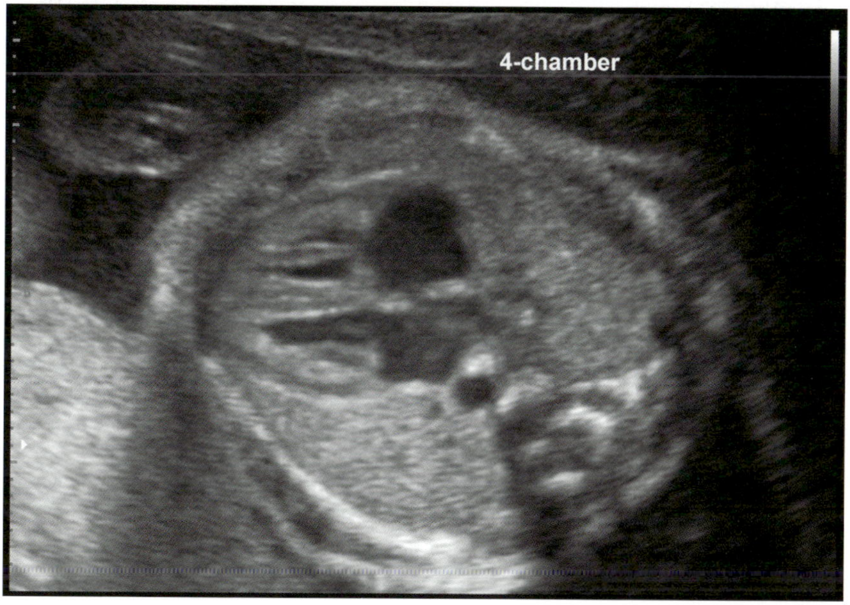

Fig. 63

2. These views provide a detailed anatomic evaluation of the spatial relationship of cardiac chambers and are also useful in the evaluation of ventricular size, ventricular wall, and septal thickness (Fig. 64).

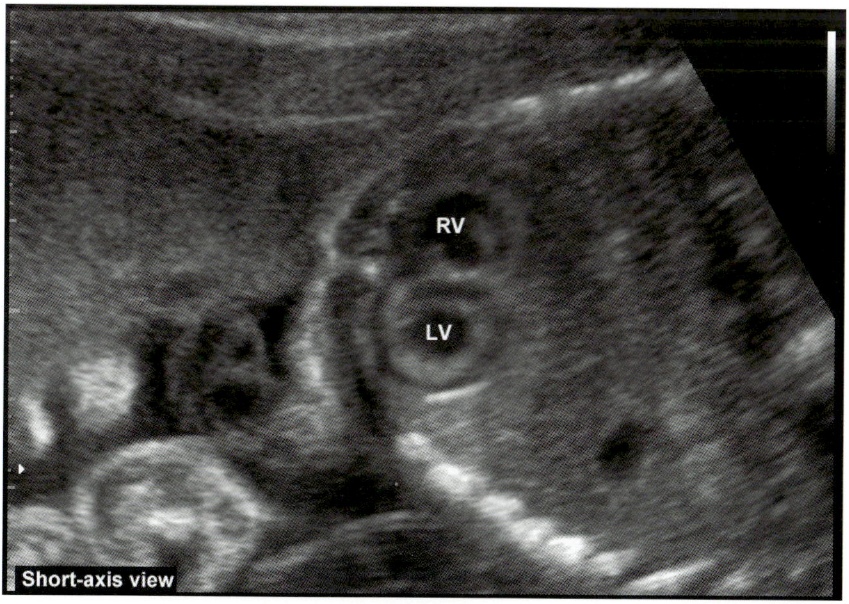

Fig. 64

3. In the apical short-axis view, the left ventricle is circular in shape and posterior to the right ventricle (Fig. 65).

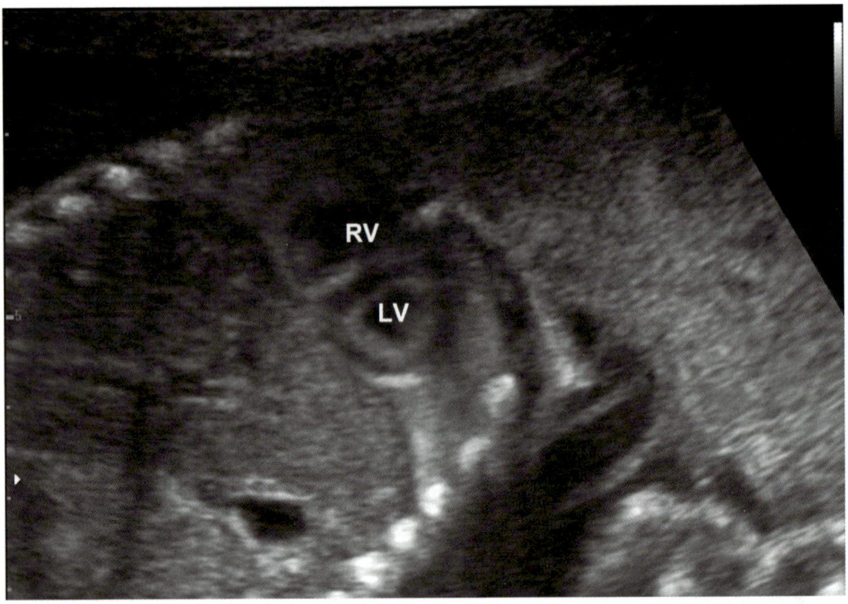

Fig. 65

9

Summary

This chapter is a quick check on what you should see to call it a normal fetal heart (Figs 1 to 11).

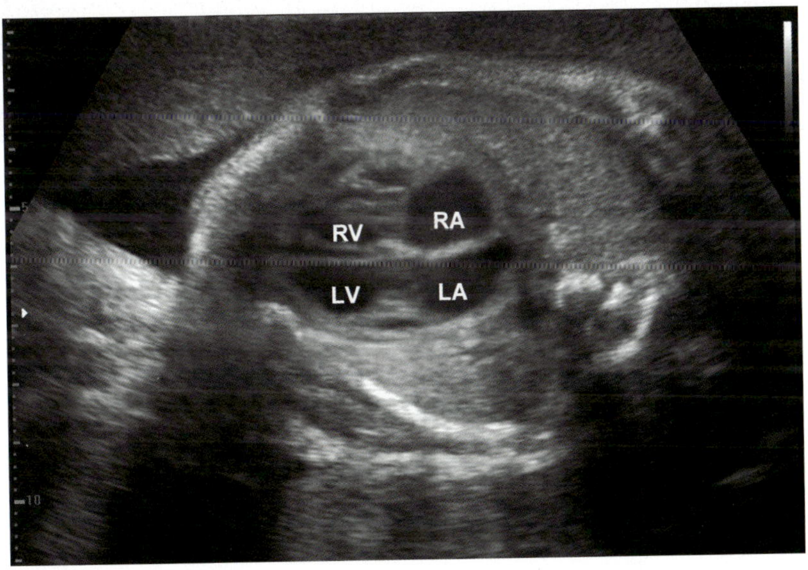

Fig. 1

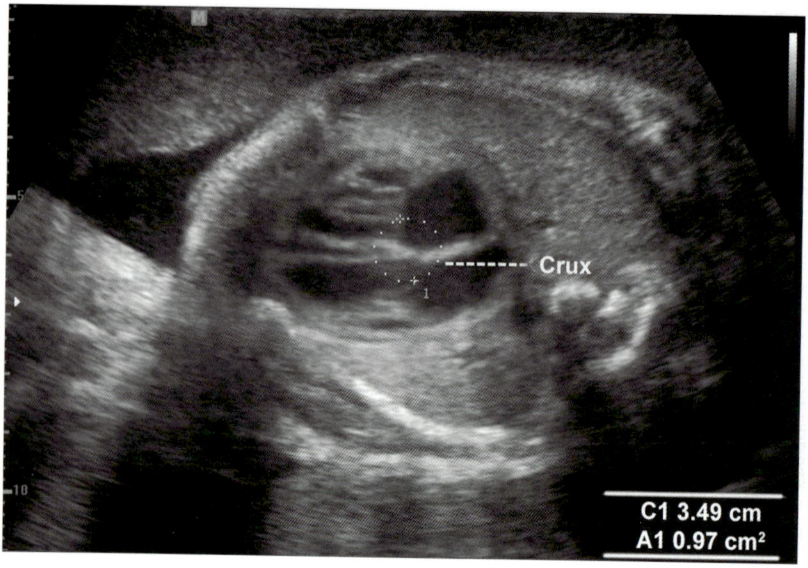

Fig. 2

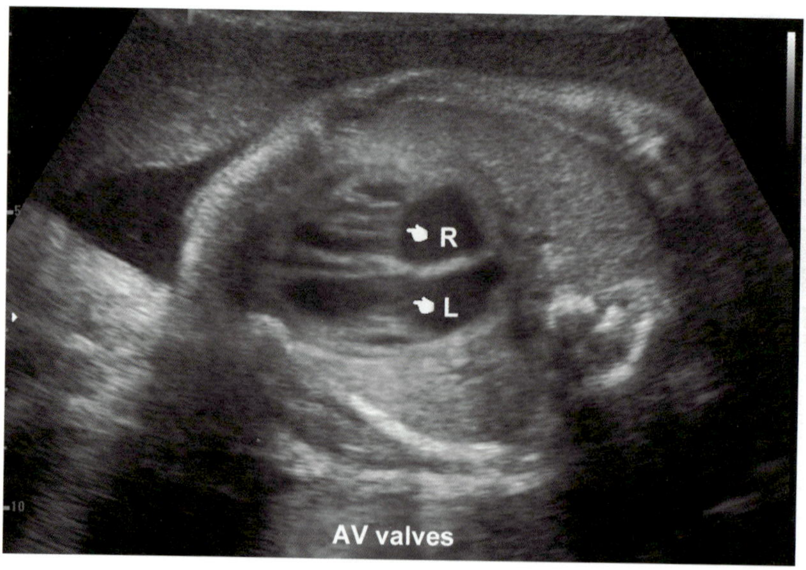

Fig. 3

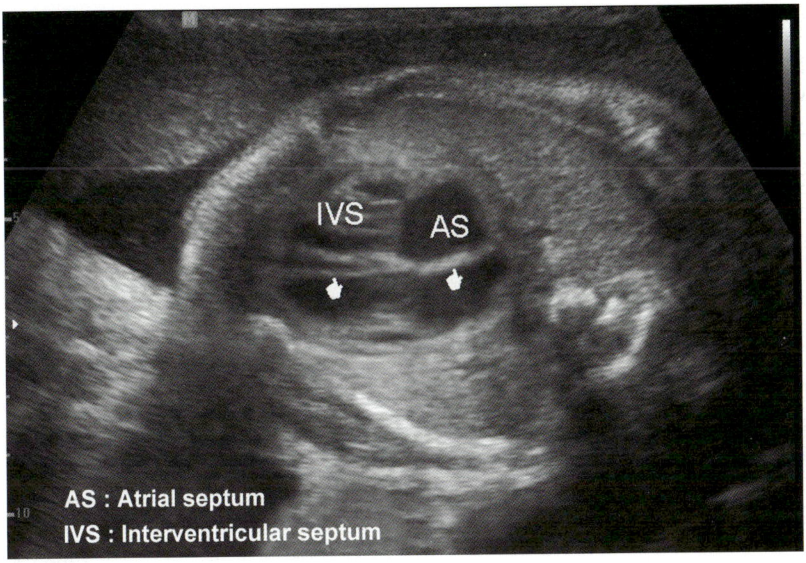
IVS
AS
AS : Atrial septum
IVS : Interventricular septum

Fig. 4

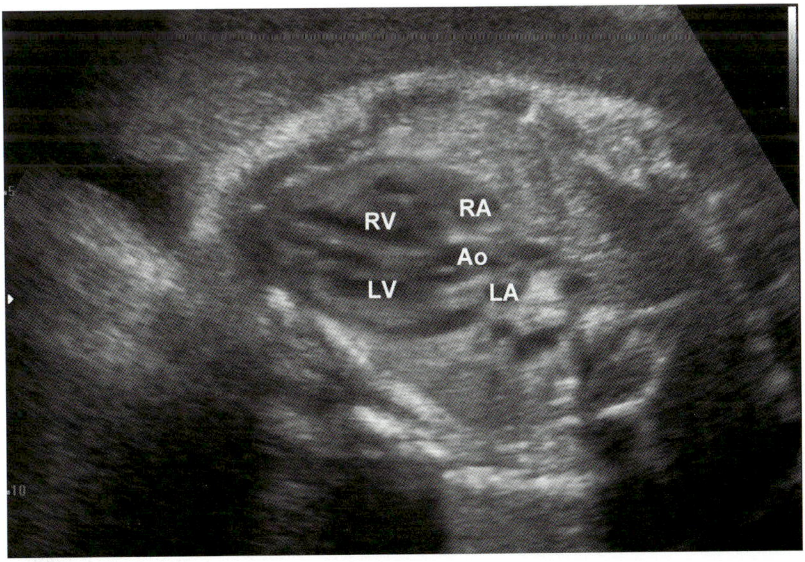
RV
RA
Ao
LV
LA

Fig. 5

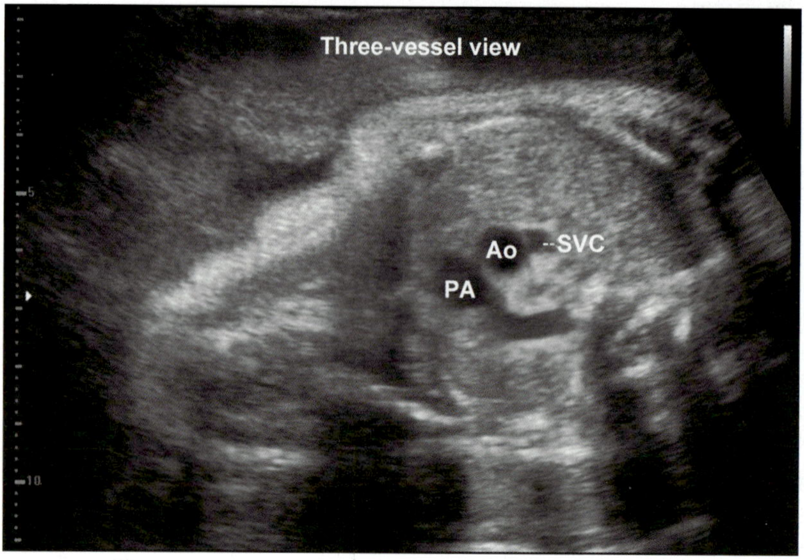

Fig. 6

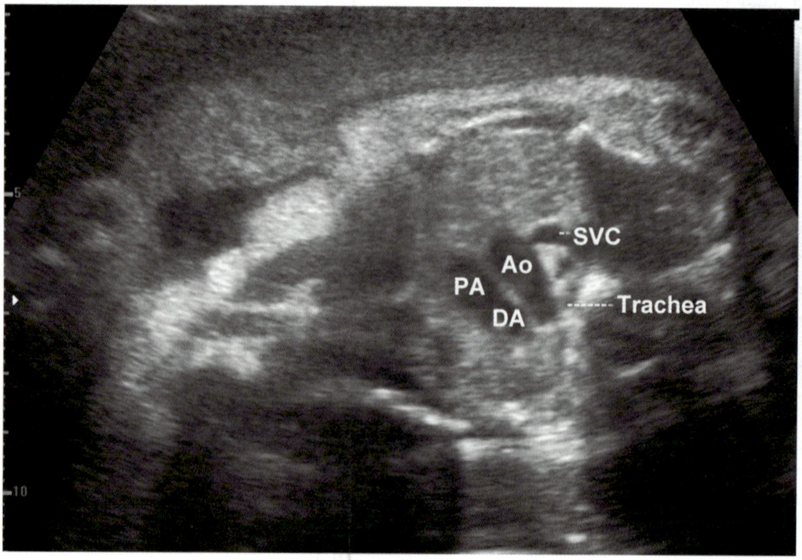

Fig. 7

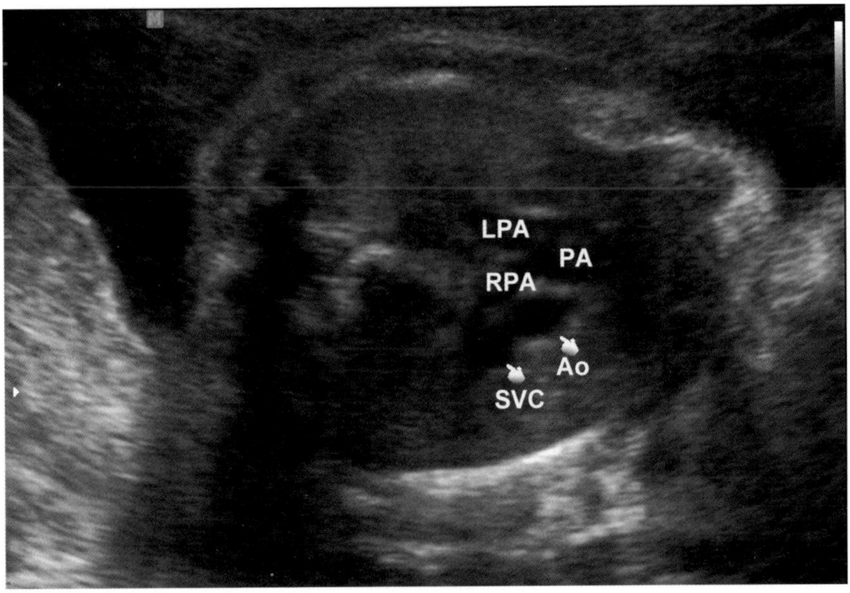

Fig. 8

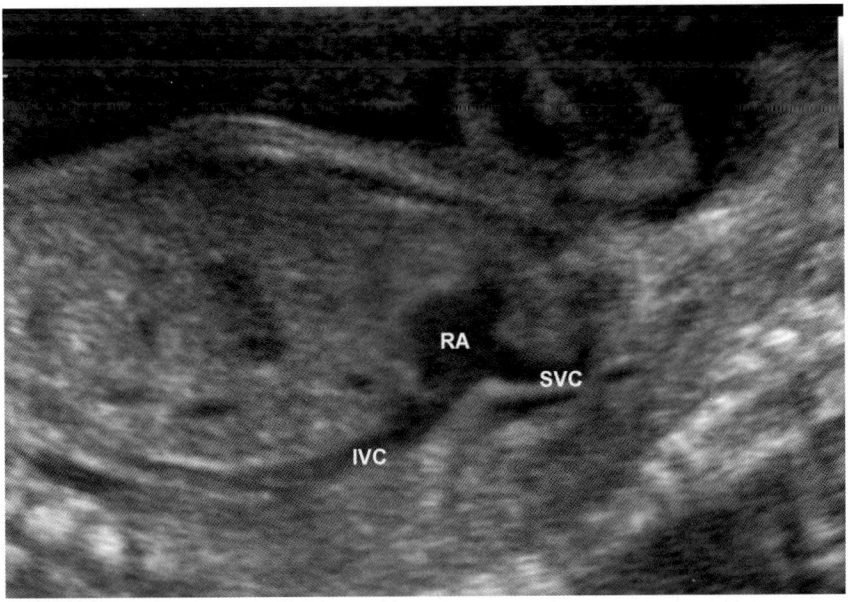

Fig. 9

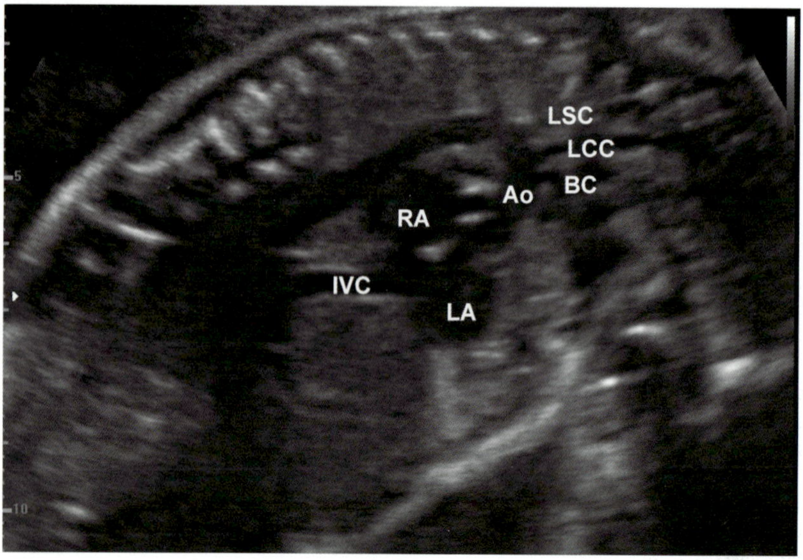
LSC
LCC
BC
Ao
RA
IVC
LA

Fig. 10

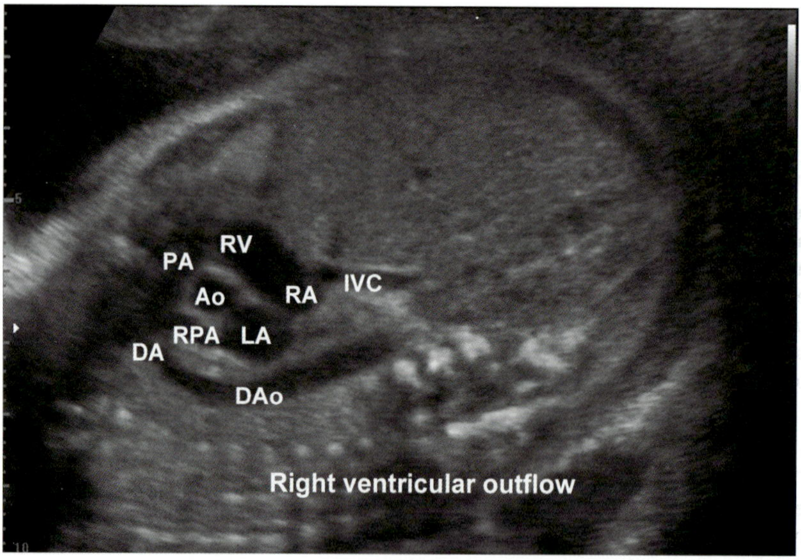
RV
PA
Ao
RA
IVC
RPA
LA
DA
DAo
Right ventricular outflow

Fig. 11

Index

P

R

S

T

V